D0580157

Modern Pilates

'This is smart exercise for people who want to know how their bodies really work and how to get the most out of them. Instead of the mindless repetitions in the gym, which in my experience only seemed to reinforce bad physical habits, Penny's teaching of Pilates has helped me to retrain, balance and strengthen my body.' *Miranda Otto, actor*

'Penny Latey's *Modern Pilates* is wonderfully comprehensive. As I continue to enjoy the life-enhancing benefits of Pilates, this remarkably detailed and thoughtful text provides me with a deeper understanding of its techniques, history and philosophy.' *Ian Cleworth, Percussionist Sydney Symphony, Synergy and TaikOz*

'Penny's incredible knowledge of anatomy is apparent in this informative book, and she imparts that wisdom generously to her readers. I have personally benefited tremendously from the instruction of Penny Latey's Modern Pilates technique which enabled me to return to professional dancing after sustaining a serious knee injury. I look forward to maintaining my muscular strength by continuing the exercises I found in *Modern Pilates*.' *Andrea Briody, dancer with Sydney Dance Company*

'Penny Latey has managed to compress her formidable knowledge of Pilates rehabilitation into a timely and accessible book . . . she manages to combine original insight into exercise therapy with a solid understanding of the traditional aspects of the Pilates system. We have had to wait some time for the genuine article on this often-misunderstood subject. It was worth the wait!' *Graham Sanders, Osteopath, B.App.Sc.(Osteo), M.Med.Sc(Clin. Epid)*

'This book is "food for thought", enquiring and encouraging us to enquire. *Modern Pilates* stands way out in front of what has been written to explain and record the method. This is a book I recommend to those who know nothing about Pilates and to those who know a lot.' *Dorothy Curnow, Pilates Practitioner*

Penelope Latey has a background in both classical and modern dance and has many years' experience in the Pilates Method, both as a dancer and for rehabilitation. She has been practising the Pilates Method for over 22 years and teaching it for 20, with a successful studio in St Leonards, Sydney. She has studied the method in London and America as well as in Australia, has been involved in training Pilates teachers for ten years and is an examiner for the Australian Pilates Method Association, for which she was the inaugural President. As well as running her busy practice and presenting professional workshops and lectures, she is also the Course Coordinator and Senior Lecturer at UTS in the Pilates Method Instructor's graduate certificate.

Modern Pilates
The step by step, at home guide
to a stronger body

Penelope Latey

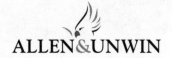

ALLEN&UNWIN

First published in Australia in 2001

Allen & Unwin
83 Alexander Street
Crows Nest NSW 2065
Australia
Phone: (61 2) 8425 0100
Fax: (61 2) 9906 2218
Email: info@allenandunwin.com
Web: www.allenandunwin.com

National Library of Australia
Cataloguing-in-Publication entry:

Latey, Penny.
   Modern pilates: the step by step, at home guide to
   a stronger body.
   Bibliography
   Includes index.

   ISBN 1 86508 598 7.

   1. Pilates method. I. Title

 613.71

Internal photography Dave Bredeson
Line illustrations Ian Faulkner 2001
Typeset in 11pt Rotis Serif by Midland Typesetters, Maryborough, Victoria
Printed by McPherson's Printing Group

10 9 8 7 6 5 4 3 2

Contents

Preface

I discovered the benefits of the Pilates method of exercise in London in the late 1970s while I was attending contemporary dance classes at 'The Place'. The problems caused by the various injuries I had sustained in my earlier years of classical ballet training, and the need to strengthen and improve flexibility in my back, led me to the basement of 'The Place' where Alan Herdman had been running a Pilates studio since he brought the method back from America in the early 1970s. The dancers at 'The Place', home of the London Contemporary Dance Company and the School of Contemporary Dance, regularly used this studio when working on a technical fault or when injured. By the time I started there, Alan's first colleague Dreas Reyneke had left to open his own studio at Notting Hill Gate and Gordon Thompson was his new assistant.

There was a strange collection of equipment squashed into a small dank space in the basement with the only natural light coming from pavement glass. The room held a sliding bed—called a universal reformer—and some raised benches, one with four posts and springs, foam shapes and light weights. The Pilates method was very hard work for me at first, but I enjoyed thinking about my body while I was trying to work on specific muscle imbalances. I also enjoyed the ability to keep exercising even when I had an injury.

For health reasons I gave up dancing early in 1980, but due to my partner's friendship with Dreas Reyneke continued doing Pilates at Dreas's Body Conditioning Studio in Notting Hill Gate, where Dreas had begun developing his own style of Pilates. Dreas has a special personality that is calm, quiet but definite. Originally a schoolteacher, he had been a dancer with Ballet Rambert for many years before taking up Pilates. I decided that I too wanted to teach Pilates.

I continued practising vigorous Pilates right up to the birth of my first child. I was still working out very strenuously as I grew larger in pregnancy and eventually had some trouble with non-expansion of abdominal muscles. After the birth of my first child I realised how much traditional Pilates focused on constantly holding in the lower abdomen and on extremely effortful movements with extreme range. The traditional method was very helpful for ultra-fit dancers and gymnasts but seemed out of tune with good function of the normal healthy body.

I began modifying the method in line with these insights. This included relaxing the constant very strong hold on flat abdominals and flat back and changing and broadening the centre to start at the pelvic floor and move up to the lower ribs. A family history of foot problems and personal experience of some post-natal incontinence problems led to my including exercises for the pelvic floor and feet as well. Not long afterwards I started teaching mat classes for pregnant and post-natal women based on these modifications.

While my training in the Pilates method was solid, through apprenticeship classes and discussions with Dreas, I began to feel I needed a better understanding of the body and undertook an anatomy, physiology and massage course. Gradually my approach to Pilates changed, and I continue to make adaptations today.

In 1988 we moved to Australia. I was extremely ill for over a year and did not go back to teaching Pilates until 1989 when I started basic mat classes at a yoga centre, then advanced Pilates classes at a professional ballet school. Shortly afterward I started my own small Pilates studio. I also became a fitness leader.

I continue to study anatomy books and occasionally do contemporary dance classes as well as regular Pilates classes. I keep up to date with developments in other movement systems. My husband Phil is an osteopath and has been a great influence and help to me. He had also done some Pilates with Dreas in London.

In 1993 I went to America on a study tour as I had by this time been teaching my own English brand of the Pilates method for more than ten years and felt I needed to look at other instructors' interpretations to refresh my understanding. Later that year I got together with a small group of Australian Pilates method instructors organised by Megan Williams and helped develop the first independent association for Pilates method instructors in Australia.

I was elected inaugural President of the Australian Pilates Method Association in 1996, retiring from that position in 1999. I have been involved with teacher training courses for Pilates method instructors since 1992, in both course development and lecturing. I continue to be involved in professional development and have been the driving force behind the new Graduate Certificate in the Pilates method at the University of Technology in Sydney. I am currently the subject coordinator and senior lecturer.

Modern Pilates is firmly based on the functional movement possibilities of the body with a solid foundation in movement anatomy. I have been influenced by contemporary dance, developments in therapeutic massage, counselling, osteo-pathy and the Feldenkrais method, Butoh (a Japanese performance art developed in the 1950s), ante- and post-natal work, my Pilates method colleagues and the problems of rehabilitation. My understanding of the method is founded on con-tinual acute examination of the body when it is moving.

Professional Associations

Australian Pilates Method Association
PO Box 1348
Crows Nest NSW 1585
Phone: (02) 9990 3021

Training Course
Enrolment enquiries for the
Graduate Certificate in the Pilates Method
Contact Denise Edwards
Unit Coordinator
University Technology Sydney (UTS)
Ultimo Campus (02) 9514 2489

Pilates Method Alliance (USA based)
www.info@pilatesmethodalliance.org

The Pilates Foundation (UK based)
www.pilatesfoundation.com

Part I

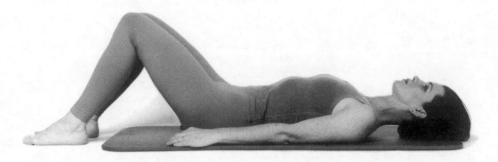

What is Pilates?

Until the mid-1980s the Pilates method of exercise was little known outside the world of dance, but it has grown in popularity rapidly in the last decade and has come out of obscurity. This section traces its history.

1 Joseph Pilates 1880–1967

Joe Pilates ran an exercise studio in New York from the late 1920s to the 1960s. He wrote two books on his method, and some films of his work are available, but otherwise his method has been passed down via apprenticeship training from teachers who were themselves apprenticed to him. It has been said that Joe did and Clara, his wife, explained. He had no formally structured teacher-training course and it is only since the 1980s that there has been any more formalised dissemination of his work. First came the book *The Pilates Method of Mental and Physical Conditioning* by P. Friedman and G. Eisen, published in 1980. Later on a number of Pilates associations and other groups of Pilates instructors around the world produced training courses of varying length, quality and depth.

This book is designed to explain some of the background to my re-interpretation of the Pilates method: placing the method firmly in the twenty-first century with our better understanding of the human body and how it functions. The Pilates method is much more than a list of exercises. It is a way of connecting and conditioning the whole being, body and mind together.

Joseph Hubertus Pilates was born in 1880 near Dusseldorf in Germany. He was apparently a sickly child, suffering from rickets, asthma and rheumatic fever. There was concern at one time that he might have tuberculosis. He was probably taken to health spas and given exercise regimes that were popular at the time for people in poor health. Long before the advent of antibiotics and other successful drugs, and the life-saving procedures of modern medicine, to stay alive meant one had to remain fit and strong, and regular exercise was one of the few ways available to combat ill health. Health spas and exercising for health had become a common part of European life.

The industrial revolution had brought more sedentary life styles and an increased density of living which led in turn to increases in contagious diseases and infant mortality, together with a general decline in health. Exercise for health was gradually introduced to the German population through the development of gymnastics. Modern gymnastics, derived from ancient Greek gymnastics, were developed by the German Ludwig Jahn early in the nineteenth century. His system started with a programme of outdoor exercise and later progressed to the use of the equipment he developed. The aim was to improve fitness and strength, primarily for men. Jahn had studied theology, history and philosophy at university and linked fitness with national pride and well-being. At the same time, Per Henrik Ling in Sweden developed another form of gymnastics (Gymnastik) emphasising rhythm and fluidity of movement. (This came to be called callisthenics, or physical education in America.) *Gymnastik* was primarily intended for women. Promoted from the late nineteenth century as a way of improving strength, endurance, flexibility and coordination, it aimed to augment the body's general well-being by placing controllable, regular demands on the cardiovascular system with coordinated breathing. Both forms of exercise became so popular that they were included in the normal curriculum in many German schools before the turn of the century. The re-introduction of gymnastics for the 1896 Olympic Games undoubtedly provided an extra boost.

The young Pilates worked so hard at improving his fitness, and at body-building, that by fourteen years of age his muscles were so clearly defined that he was posing for anatomy charts. As a teenager he enjoyed diving, skiing and gymnastics. Eventually he became a professional boxer and taught self-defence. His work in the field of exercise led him to an interest in yoga, karate, Zen meditation and the exercise regimes of the ancient Greeks and Romans.

In 1912, at the age of 32, Pilates went to England, where he worked variously as a boxer, a circus performer and a self-defence instructor. At the outbreak of World War I he was interned as an enemy alien. In camp he refined his ideas about health and body-building and encouraged all camp members to participate in his conditioning programme based on a series of exercises performed on a mat. Apparently during the influenza pandemic of 1918 no one in the internment camp died from the disease—this was considered extraordinary. Many more thousands died in that epidemic than lost their lives in the Great War.

Towards the end of the war Pilates was transferred to the Isle of Man, where he applied his knowledge to help rehabilitate the war injured. Here Pilates began experimenting with bed springs, attaching them to the ends of the beds to allow the patients to work with resistance while still bed-bound. He had realised that doing exercise with resistance helped patients recover muscle tone more quickly. This later led to his development of the 'cadillac', a four-posted bed with various springs and hanging bars, and the 'universal reformer', a sliding platform with springs on which the patient/client lies down, sits or stands. The removal of the fight against gravity in the supine position allows tension to be regulated and the spine and pelvis to be aligned. His work expanded to include various other pieces of apparatus, which in turn inspired additional mat exercises.

After the war Pilates returned to Hamburg in Germany where he refined his equipment and methods. During this time he met Rudolph Laban, the originator of Labanotation, the most widely used form of dance notation. This was Pilates' introduction to dance. Later the dance world was to be an area of fruitful cross-fertilisation for Pilates. At the same time *Gymnastik*, or physical education, was developing, with Bess Mensendieck in Hamburg and Hede Kallmeyer in Berlin both training teachers. With the release in 1925 in Germany of a film on *Gymnastik*, this more gentle form of physical education with breathing and movement gained a broader public profile.

Pilates migrated to the United States of America in 1926, a time when many Germans fled the country. His success as a self-defence instructor had attracted the attention of the German Army and it had requested his services as a trainer, a request which Pilates did not wish to respond to. Another factor contributing to his decision to migrate is believed to be his work with Max Schmeling, the German boxer. Max began his career in the early 1920s, becoming the European light-heavyweight champion in 1927–28. It is believed he had trained with Pilates. Max became German heavyweight champion in February 1928, then left for America to become world heavyweight champion in 1932. Schmeling's manager apparently helped fund Pilates' studio on 8th Avenue in New York so that the boxer could continue training with him.

On the boat to America Pilates met his future wife Clara, a nurse, who would work with him at the studio. Calling his exercise method 'Contrology', Pilates established his American studio just before the beginning of the Great Depression. There is no information on how the Depression affected the studio but in 1934 he was able to publish a small book about his method. *Your Health* sets out his philosophy and ideas about good health and how to achieve it. This little publication exudes an element of determination and frustration. Pilates refers to the 'piling up [of] fortunes, during and after the first world war . . . and the neglected . . . . necessary time to safeguard health'. The 'balance of body and mind', he claims, is the only route to good sustainable health. He goes on to deplore some of the common practices of the day in regard to looking after babies and children. He explains the roots of ill health from childhood onwards as poor care and lack of exercise. Towards the end his booklet becomes a long advertising essay espousing his method of exercise, good hygiene, and explaining why one should use his specially designed beds and chairs that are 'posturally correct'. He ends by voicing his dismay that some of his advice and work is used without due acknowledgement, something the Pilates community still has problems with today.

Even though Pilates had experience with strength and fitness training, gymnastics, boxing, and instructing for self-defence, in the long term it was dancers who worked with him most enthusiastically. Pilates became a close friend of Ted Shawn, a dancer who, with Ruth St Denis, founded the Denis-Shawn Dance Company, then went on to help develop the dance centre at Jacob's Pillow in the mid-1930s. Ted welcomed many different forms of movement, and Joe taught mat classes and outdoor training there. Ron Fletcher was one of the first well-known dancers to use contrology. Pilates' ability to return dancers to the stage after back and leg injuries gained him an excellent relationship in the dance world with people like Hanya Holm, Martha Graham and the choreographer George Balanchine, who all recommended him. By the end of the 1940s he had developed a significant clientele among dancers.

Pilates' second book, *Return to Life Through Contrology*, written with W. J. Miller, was published in 1945. In it he sets out the development of his philosophy and a list of exercises to follow and practise at home. He wrote no other books.

By the time Pilates died in 1967, a number of studios based on his method had been opened, catering to its extensive following in the American dance world. During this time Clara had worked side by side with Joe and after his death continued to run the studio until her own death in 1977.

Pilates was extremely possessive of his method of exercise; even though he taught about half a dozen instructors, he was reluctant to entrust it to others and remained the sole master at his studio. Except for *Your Health* and *Return to Life Through Contrology*, nothing comprehensive was published about his method until after he and Clara had died. In 1980 *The Pilates Method of Physical and Mental Conditioning*, written by P. Friedman and G. Eisen, was published. This book clearly sets out, with some refinements, his philosophy and principles, and the mat exercises of his method.

Pilates taught his assistants by apprenticeship. His early assistants tended to move away and open their own studios, Ron Fletcher and Carola Trier among them, but some, like his later assistant Romana Kryzanowski, stayed with him. Eve Gentry, another early apprentice, moved away to pursue dance then returned to the method, bringing with her clearly organised, gentle exercises called pre-Pilates and a new approach to some of the principles. Some of Pilates' early followers merged his work with their own, and some students took pieces of the method, sometimes only the exercises without understanding the principles, and developed their own style, though still labelling it 'Pilates'. There are consequently many different interpretations of the Pilates method, each subtly altered by new understandings of the human body or influenced by one of the many new movement styles that were developed from the beginning of the twentieth century.

Today, not only dancers and athletes use the Pilates method extensively; with modifications and variations to some of the exercises, but the general public is beginning to use it for post-acute rehabilitation and for general fitness.

2 Traditional Pilates philosophy and principles

The exercise system which Joseph Pilates developed mixed the practical movement styles and ideas of gymnastics, martial arts, yoga and dance with philosophical notions. Pilates was a great reader and was fond of quoting the German philosophers, F. von Schiller ('It is the mind itself which shapes the body') and Arthur Schopenhauer ('To neglect one's body for any other advantage in life is the greatest follies [sic]'), two principles he incorporated into his beliefs.

This amalgamation of philosophy and exercise (movement) and the performing arts has been common in Germany from the nineteenth century onwards.

Pilates was only one of a number of Europeans to develop and interrelate the concepts of physical practice and mental discipline.

Pilates' 1934 booklet *Your Health* was produced by the 'Prof. Pilates Health Studios'. In the Introduction he said:

> PERFECT *Balance of Body and Mind, is that quality in civilised man, which not only gives him superiority over the savage and animal kingdom, but furnishes him with all the physical and mental powers that are dispensable for attaining the goal of Mankind—HEALTH and HAPPINESS.*
>
> *The purpose of this booklet is to transmit in a simple form, the course of present day ill-health and immoral conditions, and the resultant effects which prevent the average human being from attaining this physical perfection—man's inherited birthright.*

Knowing Pilates' background one can understand much of his determined belief in the rightness of his method. He berates the 'quack' cures promoted by 'proprietors of patent medicines and manufacturers of mechanical apparatus, massaging belts, rowing machines, nostrums, serums and other injections', possibly referring to other early exercise regimes, patent cure-alls from 'snake oil' salesmen and early forms of unsuccessful innoculations. He believed that wellness began in childhood and that 'The first lesson is correct breathing ... properly instructed how to draw the abdomen in and out at the same time holding their breath for a short time. Then they should also learn how to fully deflate the lungs in exhaling'.

The remarkable health sustained by the detainees in the internment camp during World War I, especially in the face of the influenza pandemic, and the consequences of the use of mustard gas, plus his own asthma and the prevalence of tuberculosis, all things that affect the lungs, must have focused Pilates' mind on breathing problems. He was probably also aware of Leo Kofler, the Delsarte system and Else Gindler and her followers, whose systems worked with breathing.

Pilates felt most people were overdressed and overheated and did not wash properly. On hygiene: '"Hardening" of the body ... fewer clothes the better ...

Cleanliness of the skin . . . massaging with brush'. Does this hark back to his early childhood when he was improving his health?

On posture and breathing: 'Drawing in of stomach and the throwing out of the chest . . . the spine of every normal child is straight. The back is perfectly flat'. Pilates believed that a healthy adult should also have a flat spine. Overweight problems, particularly around the abdomen, 'have their origin in the "miss-carriage" of the spine' and poor posture affects good health.

There were no exercise descriptions in *Your Health*, however. Pilates most definitely wanted clients to attend his studio. Around this time Pilates drew up designs for a bed and chairs. These were never manufactured, though his Wunda chair (which he made himself), is of similar design to his armchair. I do think that Pilates had a point about the quality of chair design, and problems associated with spending hours sitting.

Eleven years later he published *Return to Life Through Contrology* (hereafter referred to as *Return to Life*), written with W. J. Millar. In this 1945 book, Pilates describes his work as 'Contrology', sets out the philosophy behind his work and, for the first time, describes (briefly) and illustrates a series of 34 exercises to do at home. The explanation of the philosophy that underpins his exercise system is more comprehensive.

'Contrology is complete co-ordination of body, mind, and spirit.' I think Pilates has added spirit to his earlier definition, so that his method more fully encompasses the whole person, including their emotional wellbeing. 'Control-ogy restores physical fitness . . . [it] develops the body uniformly, corrects wrong postures, restores physical vitality, invigorates the mind, and elevates the spirit. It makes you feel good and gives you "all-confidence".' His guiding prin-ciples included 'concentrating on the purpose of the exercises as you performed them'.

Pilates enlarges on his ideas about correct breathing in *Return to Life*:

> *The exercises . . . stirred your sluggish circulation into action and to performing its duty more effectively in the matter of discharging through the bloodstream the accumulation of fatigue-products created by muscular and mental activities. Your brain clears and your will power functions.*

He believed that vigorous exercise was important, as this achieved a 'bodily house-cleaning with blood circulation', and that breathing correctly helped your body remove harmful germs. 'True heart control follows correct breathing which simultaneously reduces heart strain, purifies the blood, and develops the lungs.' Pilates felt it was vital to breathe both deeply and fully: 'Squeeze every atom of air from your lungs until they are almost as free of air as is a vacuum'.

Stretching and rolling the spine (with the chin pressed tightly to the chest) was also important; this helped to correct posture by flattening out the curves in the spine and straightening out the body. Pilates believed that the back should be flat 'like a plumb line' (like a baby's), thus in performing floor exercises, the full length of the back was always pressed firmly against the mat. Pilates also thought that one always had to articulate or move evenly throughout the spine, and that one needed to exercise *all* the muscles: 'Developing minor muscles naturally helps to strengthen major muscles'.

The exercises were described in detail, with breathing movements and aim carefully noted, and illustrated with many photos. Words commonly used in describing how to do the exercises include 'keep legs (tensed, knees locked)' . . . 'arms rigid, shoulders locked' . . . 'fists clenched' . . . 'snap-kick'. Films which show Pilates working and teaching reveal his extreme vigour and fast dynamics, matching his written descriptions of how to move. These facts, and his very definite philosophy, suggest that he was a very robust man physically and mentally and that to even attempt his original exercises one would have to be equally robust.

After Pilates and Clara's deaths, his method, as described by Friedman and Eisen in 1980 in *The Pilates Physical and Mental Conditioning*, subtly changed. The fundamental principles remained the same, but new ones were added, and the original principles more clearly delineated. Most importantly, the concept of 'centre' which Pilates called the 'powerhouse', was named and carefully explained. The range of exercises was enlarged and developed, with exercises structured into progressive levels. The traditional approach of all-out effort and extreme vigour was relaxed slightly, while still retaining a dynamic approach to movement.

Development has continued since then, and there are now what are termed 'pre-Pilates exercises' as well as a whole range of Pilates-based exercises with further variations and modifications. Some of the exercises have been simplified to ensure connection with the body from the inside out, making the method more accessible. The principles have been refined to reflect current understanding of applied anatomy, physiology and kinesiology.

3 Developments of the traditional principles

In the 1970s and early 1980s, many more Pilates studios opened in America, and the method went offshore when Alan Herdman brought it to London and started his studio at 'The Place'. Although still only taught by apprenticeship, the method was now influenced by Friedman and Eisen's clear descriptions of how to exercise correctly by following six fundamental principles.

Concentration: *To do the movements properly, you must pay attention to what you are doing . . . No part of your body is unimportant; no motion can be ignored. ('You have to concentrate on what you are doing. All the time.')*
Control: *The reason you need to concentrate so thoroughly is so you can be in Control of every aspect of every movement. Not just the large motions of your limbs but the positions of your fingers, head and toes, the degree of arch or flatness of your back, the rotation of your wrists, the turning in or out of your legs.*
Centering: *'Our first requirement in concentrating on our bodies and gaining full control of them is a starting place: somewhere to begin building our own bodily foundation.*

Consider the part of your body that forms a continuous band, front and back, between the bottom of your rib cage and the line across your hip bones. We call this your "center"; . . . the center is the focal point of the Pilates Method.
Flowing movement: *Nothing should be stiff or jerky. Nothing should be too rapid or too slow. Smoothness and evenly flowing movement go hand in hand with control.*
Precision: *Concentrate on right movements each time you exercise,*

. . . else you will do them improperly and lose their value', (Pilates stated).

Breathing*: Full and thorough inhalation and exhalation are part of every Pilates exercise. Joe saw forced exhalation as the key to full inhalation. 'Squeeze out the lungs as you would wring out a wet towel . . . soon the entire body is charged with fresh oxygen from toes to fingertips' . . . [Romana Kryzanowska and many other American Pilates method teachers use] . . . 'breathe in on the point of effort and out on the return or relaxation. . . .' [The other rule is] If you are doing something that squeezes your body tight, use the motion to squeeze air out of your lungs and inhale when you straighten up.*

So concentrating, controlling movement, coordinating full and deep breathing and centring the body in order to move with an economy of effort are crucial aspects of the method. The quality of each movement is emphasised rather than encouraging mindless repetition. By avoiding strain or pain through attention to detail, precision and flow of movement is sustained. Breathing is an important element of the method, both to heighten breathing awareness, to help focus and use the centre and to increase oxygen intake.

Freidman and Eisen also describe ways of 'finding' the body. In discussing relaxation, for example, they note that because there is an emphasis on control, concentration and precision there is a tendency for clients to tense up, 'using far more effort than necessary; in essence they are over-controlling. The cure for this is to relax the muscles while maintaining enough tone to hold the position you want.'

On lengthening and strengthening they note that Pilates always wanted the client to use a full range of movement, encouraging 'lengthening out the body as you worked it'–thus the client always lengthened away from the centre. Friedman and Eisen move away from 'locking' the joints to 'straightening' and stretching out the joints 'long and thin' to find maximum extension.

Turning to the notion of the straight spine: Pilates was keen on stretching through the spine and neck. His original instructions for creating a flat back include the words 'navel to spine', 'spine to mat' and 'press the base of the skull into the mat'. Friedman and Eisen confirmed this with 'chin to chest' and 'stretching the neck', which flattens the whole spine. Getting the client 'sitting up out of your hips' continued the straight spine idea by squeezing the buttocks so tight that the thighs turn out, encouraging the pelvis to tilt posteriorly. All this aimed at creating a flat back, which we now know is not a good thing. Friedman and Eisen also included 'correct' foot positions, avoidance of hunched shoulders and articulating the spine one vertebra at a time, also controlled with pinched buttocks.

The understanding that improvements will take time, commitment and consistency, and that 'one properly done movement is worth any number of sloppy ones', is continued in their book, with the proviso that pain and strain are to be avoided.

Friedman and Eisen's principles can be summarised as concentration, control, centring, flowing movement, precision and breathing. As the first comprehensive record of the method, Pilates' own publications aside, their work is invaluable.

4 Present-day Pilates

There are now almost as many variations to the Pilates method as there are people who practise it. The different styles can be roughly divided into a few different types. Up until the end of the 1980s there were three distinct styles—American West Coast, American East Coast and British. By the early 1990s, with the profession gathering momentum, distinctions of place had changed to the broad categories of hard, soft, and rehabilitative Pilates, and Pilates-based exercises. Current styles can be divided into two basic schools—the repertory approach and modern Pilates. The repertory approach closely follows the original exercises as described by Pilates himself, and later by Friedman and Eisen. This more traditional method follows closely set exercise sequences and set numbers of repetitions, with only small adaptations and modifications for different body types or problems. It is fairly fast and dynamic right from the start of the programme. It is primarily for the completely problem-free person or those who are already trained, like dancers. The repertory approach has been exploited further, with some large Pilates mat classes being presented by people with very little training in the method. The briefness of the training courses—anything from 3–4 days to a few weekends—means that the quality of the classes can be very poor. Injury can happen if some exercises are taught out of context, and without proper guidance or attention to the principles.

Modern Pilates, on the other hand, uses Joseph Pilates' philosophy and modified principles with a more gradual introduction to the exercises, and includes adaptations and developments that connect with our improved knowledge of how the body works. It is further influenced by other movement disciplines, by developments in psychology and by theories of emotional factors and how the mind works. It is the origin of my approach. The initial emphasis here is on understanding the body and improving awareness, connecting breathing, getting the right muscles working and the over-worked areas de-stressed. Clients attending a modern-style studio have at least one or more private consultations where a posture and movement assessment is conducted and any history of injury or illness noted.

Classes are in a very small group setting with the clients working at their own pace, and individually supervised. The exercises are always tailored to the clients' particular needs, body types, weaknesses and strengths. The foundations of breathing, alignment and working from the centre are emphasised initially. A broader range of exercises is then introduced to assist in applying the principles of the method, encompassing other movement styles and gradually moving towards a more dynamic approach. Traditional exercises are utilised only when appropriate breathing, correct alignment and muscle control have become second nature to the body.

Growing interest in the Pilates method has been generated by this broadening of approach, and also by changes in the general public's need to look after themselves, not only with ageing baby boomers becoming injury-conscious in the wake of the aerobic exercise boom, but also because of the 'famous people syndrome', where those in the public eye are admitting that the Pilates method helps them look after their bodies. The modern interpretation of the method can be applied safely to both fit and unfit people, and ranges from post-trauma rehabilitation to fitness for the ordinary body to fine-tuning of elite athletes.

It is certainly easier and quicker to train teachers in the older repertory method, and large group classes lend themselves to that style—but it is only a productive approach if the client already has good body awareness and flexibility, no injuries or problems, and is happy to build strength in set areas rather than working muscles more selectively.

Steps toward modern Pilates

In America in the 1980s Eve Gentry developed and refined postural alignment and the breathing techniques set down by Joe Pilates, and connected these changes with a new way of finding the centre called imprinting. This focuses awareness on where the vertebrae of the spine are in space and in relation to the body through using the abdominals to stabilise the lower back without tucking the pelvis. This fits with the concept of the neutral spine, quite different from the flat back of the earlier approaches to posture and centred control. Eve's approach was more relaxed with the joints floating in the body (joint release) rather than being locked and compressed.

At the same time in England, new interpretations were being developed by Dreas Reyneke, Alan Herdman's first apprentice, now in his own studio. Dreas, with some input from osteopath Phil Latey and myself, introduced and encouraged natural spinal alignment, enlarged the centre to include the pelvic floor and introduced specific foot exercises.

During the 1990s many books were published, some repeating the more traditional approach found in *Return to Life* and Freidman and Eisen, others promoting modern developments. A few writers reinterpreted the original principles, adding 'relaxation', 'alignment', 'coordination' and 'stamina', removing 'precision' and 'control'. These changes partially reflect the changed perspective of modern society. The concept of control with its connotations of overpowering and forcing the body to work sensibly has been dropped. We wish to be more in tune with our body, to manage and connect with, not bully it. But other changes, it seems to me, miss the point, and new principles such as 'coordination' sometimes lack depth of explanation.

5 Traditional Pilates versus modern Pilates

Traditional or repertory Pilates closely follows the exercises set out in *Return to Life* and Friedman and Eisen.

To achieve some of the positions and range of motion expected in traditional

Pilates exercises, some muscle groups have to work very hard. In fact the muscle recruitment required for traditional Pilates tends to contradict Joe Pilates' belief in working all the muscles of the body evenly. There is also the implicit assumption that all bodies are similar in proportions to Joseph Pilates' body, thus ease of working in the traditional way is dependent on the client having a similar balance of muscle bulk, bony alignment and stature. Pilates, however, had a quite short and stocky mesomorphic body type. His centre, or powerhouse, appears to lie in the hip flexor origins and glutei muscles, the lower pelvis, buttocks and upper thighs. Proponents of traditional Pilates do tend to have very strong buttock muscles, thighs (particularly hip flexors) and powerful upper body strength, particularly across the shoulders, and large wrists. Pilates was, after all, first a boxer and gymnast. His early floor classes included standing boxing and martial arts warm-ups.

It is not surprising that Pilates valued strength and speed of movement and persistent vigorous effort, with his history of childhood illness and exercising as one of the few ways to regain health as a teenager, coupled with his early experiences as an adult. His belief that vigorous exercise with full breathing and a straight spine, light clothing, proper hygiene, moderate food intake and adequate rest was the only way to remain fit, healthy and alive was well founded.

Pilates integrated many movement methods into his own special style of exercise, which is particularly reminiscent of the early Swedish gymnastics of Per Henrik Ling. His method would have appeal for the fit but be extremely difficult for the unwell. One of the reasons the method was enthusiastically embraced by dancers was its similarity to dance in its pursuit of full to extreme range of movement with precision and control, something a dancer is always attempting to achieve.

Pilates' ability to keep the rest of an injured dancer's body very fit while allowing the injured body part to heal, thus allowing the dancer to return to performing almost as soon as the injury is repaired, remains highly relevant today and can be applied to all people of all fitness levels. Dancers need, and have, very strong buttocks, hip flexors and thighs as well as good flexibility. The focus on abdominal strength is especially appropriate for contemporary dancers.

Traditional Pilates exercises primarily work in a forward and/or back movement technically called the sagittal plane. There is little diagonal or spiral

work until   Pilates increases the
range of spiral or diagonal work, particularly in the basic and intermediate
programmes.

Pilates was very hands-on, guiding clients' bodies physically as well as
verbally. His use of touch to correct a movement was a very important part of his
work at a time when touching a client's body was relatively taboo (except in the
dance world). This was not to change till the late 1950s. The use of touch con-
tinues to be an important teaching tool in a Pilates studio, though the manner is
less forceful. Touch can improve muscle engagement and relaxation.

Despite the inflexibility of the original written programmes, Pilates did suggest
some modifications from time to time, such as repeating during the day exercises
that focused on areas of the body that needed work, and he apparently modified
and developed specific exercises for certain clients. In *Return to Life*, however, he
advised that one must always do 'the hundred', a particularly arduous exercise,
before attempting anything else. I must emphasise, however, that this exercise is
extremely dangerous for someone new to the method and, even under supervision,
can result in serious injuries (see page 198 forward for more on Pilates' original
exercises). His emphasis on quality not quantity was not always adhered to by the
profession. While Pilates thought a few well-done movements most effective,
some studios in the 1980s were insisting on 20 or more repetitions of everything.

Even up until the early 1980s Pilates studios in the UK primarily attracted
dancers as clients, but gradually members of the public were being recommended
to the studios, particularly by osteopaths. Actors, musicians and singers also
found the method useful.

In the 1990s Pilates began to be promoted to the general public for fitness,
as a safe alternative to aerobics and weight work for clients who had injured
themselves.

6   Modern Pilates fundamentals

Modern Pilates thus uses the fundamentals of Joe Pilates' work, philosophy and
exercises with modifications that make it appropriate for those of any age, for

the unwell, during p   very fit elite
athlete or dancer. I   tals and redefined them, placing them firmly in the new century.

Beginning with Joe Pilates' original words and ideas, from *Your Health* and *Return to Life*, I will show how modern fundamentals are firmly embedded in his primary, essential ideas.

> *The simplest law of nature—balance of body and mind . . .*
>
> *It is the conscious control of all muscular movements of the body. It is the correct utilisation and application of the leverage principles afforded by the bones comprising the skeletal framework of the body, a complete knowledge of the mechanism of the body, and a full understanding of the principles of the equilibrium and gravity as applied to the movements of the body in motion, at rest and sleep . . . 'Contrology'* (Your Health, *p. 20).*

Concentration

These fundamentals—first of all, 'conscious' control of the body—require thought and focused attention, a heightened awareness of the body. Concentrating on what you are going to do, and connecting the mind and body, mean that we have to tune in to our bodily sensory systems. In other words, we concentrate to bring our attention inwards in order to recognise bodily sensation accurately: achieve conscious control.

Awareness

> *Ideally, our muscles should obey our will. Reasonably, our will should not be dominated by the reflex actions of our muscles* (Return to Life, *p. 6).*

To not be dominated by unthinking reflex actions we need to be aware of our bodies, to listen to the messages sent from the body to the brain. We need knowledge and understanding to look after ourselves. The first step is *concentrating* on improving our *awareness* of those components that make up our selves, attentively thinking, feeling and consciously using our muscles, aware but not overly or consumingly conscious to achieve balance of body and mind, not domination of the body by the mind. In other words, we are talking about *focused awareness.*

Alignment

Progressing from connecting the mind's awareness of the body (and its self), Pilates' system was based on 'complete knowledge of the mechanism[s] of the body'. He expected his clients to acquire a full understanding of their internal sense of equilibrium and gravity through movement. Following through from Pilates' desire for understanding and knowledge, this book will introduce you to the anatomy and physiology of the body as it relates to movement and exercise in modern Pilates.

To apply the leverage principles afforded by the skeletal system, some understanding of the 'carriage of the body' (the body's placement in space, or postural alignment) is necessary. Understanding one's individual optimal postural alignment (neutral posture) will allow economy of movement, a natural flow of compensatory patterns, so that no muscle is overworked or misused, without aiming for perfect symmetry.

Breathing

> *Before any real benefit can be derived from physical exercises, one must first learn how to breathe properly . . . Our very life depends on it* (Your Health, *p. 42).*

Pilates felt that correct breathing would 'accomplish more toward attaining and maintaining maximum health standards, than all other remedies', that correct breathing would 'bring practically every other muscle of the entire system into play' and that this would allow our posture to be 'normal'. Pilates' ideas on how to breathe were somewhat extreme in today's terms, however, and the method up until recently focused on lateral breathing, using primarily the lower ribs.

Modern Pilates does emphasise breathing with the movements and, most importantly *not* holding one's breath, and refines the breath work. Conscious breath work not only distributes aerobic muscle food to the body, it also allows us to connect with our internal bodily functions. It is a physical interface between the outside and inside of the body, increasing awareness and encouraging proper torso control of the centre with the use of lower ribs and abdominal muscles, improving alignment and promoting internal relaxation.

Centring

The *centre*, so-named by Friedman and Eisen, was referred to by Pilates as the powerhouse of the body. Up until recently the centre referred to the area from the hips to the lower ribs but the modern centre has been redefined. Today, working from the centre means working the muscles that travel from the pelvic floor to the thoracic diaphragm, not just sucking in and holding the stomach and overusing buttock and hip flexors. Working from the centre also interconnects with proper shoulder support. The deep postural muscles of the whole torso are retrained first, thus freeing up the movements of the limbs. Centring is pivotal to the practice of Pilates, as it initiates economic and graceful movement.

Having established these foundations, how do we move and perform the exercises?

Precision

To improve the quality of our movement our ability to be precise is employed. Precision is vital for retraining the body's postural alignment. Specific muscle control and much closer mental connection (neuro-muscular patterning) are developed with increased precision. Precise thinking leads to precise movement, thus conserving momentum with no impact or loss of balance. Fine motor control contributes to separating moving (locomotor) functions from supporting (stabilising) functions through natural alignment—turning on the little-used muscles, turning down the overused muscles. Listening to the feedback that we get from our body sensors (proprioceptors) makes us aware of what we are doing. Precision assists coordination; it is the practical application of awareness.

Coordination

Coordination is defined in the *Shorter Oxford Dictionary*, in terms of physiology, as 'the combined action of a number of muscles in the production of certain complex movements'.

Pilates states, 'vitality [of the body] is dependent on the absolute coordination of the body and mind—perfect balance' (*Your Health*, p. 20).

Coordination creates the possibility of *flowing movement* and smooth transitions from one action to the next. For me, it is the unconscious grasp of complex sequentiality in fine muscle action to create flowing, global, emotionally connected whole body movements.

Complex movements require more than just strength in forward and back movement, they require movement ability in all spatial directions. Modern Pilates increases the degree of multiplanar action in proper coordination, requiring a lot more work in diagonal and spiral movements, while sustaining equilibrium via use of the aligned centre.

Lengthening

Lengthening as you work helps with both centring and alignment. To elongate the body as you exercise refines its coordination. Most importantly, Pilates incorporated this principle of lengthening into all his exercises. Lengthening encourages two important aspects of the Pilates method. Firstly, stretching the muscles to full range requires muscle balance, with the muscles lengthening and working at the same time (eccentric work) with proper support from the centre. Second, as the body lengthens the diagonally opposed supporting muscles have to work well. Most other exercise methods focus on the shortening muscle work and ignore the complex role of the supporting muscles.

Pilates again: 'True flexibility is achieved only when all muscles are uniformly developed.'

His original exercises were meant to provide flexibility. Certainly, some do improve flexibility if one already has a good range of movement, but for many people good flexibility needs to start in a gentler place. For most untrained bodies the action of sitting upright with the legs straight in front is, frankly, impossible. Many modern instructors incorporate gentle, slow and thoughtful stretches in their classes—this is very important, as muscles do not lengthen or stretch out by themselves. I assume that Pilates' lack of easier stretches was at least in part due to the fact that he had many dancers as clients (dancers tend to overstretch). The focus on lengthening work increased when 'active resisted movement' exercises were incorporated into the method, thus improving the range of muscle strength and reducing joint compression.

Persistence

Persistence is the final principle. With consistent practice and perseverance the Pilates method helps one to acquire comfortable body alignment, good posture and fitness. Persistence here means more than stamina and endurance—it includes the determination to learn and to improve and extend our mental attention span as well as our physical abilities. Omitting this principle as some have done makes for a fairly mechanistic approach and misses the need to keep on trying mentally and psychologically as well as physically. Persistence alludes to how difficult the method can be, particularly, at the beginning. There are no quick fixes, no instant fitness, no short cuts. Without persistence one misses out on the real long-term benefits of the method, as improvements are gradual at first, building up over the years.

These principles, starting with the first and moving down sequentially, all interlock with and support each other. Modern Pilates may initially appear reductionistic but the process and interconnectedness, working the mind and body together, builds a wholeness that is more than the sum of its parts.

Pilates in action

Modern Pilates has been influenced by other movement programmes and hands-on treatment modalities such as massage, Rolfing and British osteopathy. It has also been influenced by improved understanding of anatomy and physiology, new ways of looking at injury and the process of illness, advances in medical treatment, new understandings in counselling and developments in psychology and teaching skills.

The Pilates method has itself influenced many forms of dance, movement education and therapy as well as rehabilitation methods and different types of body work. It has given physiotherapy a new direction and influenced exercise prescription in many body work fields including sports medicine. Some principles and exercises have been incorporated into modern yoga and dance, fitness training and coaching methods in some sports.

Modern Pilates can be for anyone who wants to be able to move with awareness and grace and sustain long term fitness. However, if you have any special health problems or have recently sustained an injury, doing Pilates at home with only this book as a guide is not a good idea. If you have any kind of problem please go to an accredited Pilates studio where the instructors can supervise your progress and assist you to get the right muscles moving and the wrong ones resting. Properly supervised modern Pilates is ideal for injury prevention and post-acute rehabilitation. This book will help you gain insights into how the method works and how your body works, and will help you in your practice if you already attend a Pilates studio.

Modern Pilates method is the thoughtful person's exercise method. Initially it can seem quite strange to approach movement and exercise via thinking and feeling first, but to efficiently retrain the body out of old postural habits and connect with underused muscles we need to find out what is actually happening in the body before we can start to change it.

Patiently improving body awareness and muscle connections will give long-term benefits and create a foundation on which to build towards more dynamic work without pain, injury or muscle over development. The principles can and should be applied to everyday life.

The details in the following chapters do not need to be understood straight away or all at once—we gradually improve the connection with our body and gradually improve muscle strength and flexibility. We need time to digest and understand and feel our body. Through using the basic exercises we can achieve good postural alignment and improve body awareness and connectedness. Repeating these exercises regularly will improve the ability to concentrate and think more fruitfully.

Part II

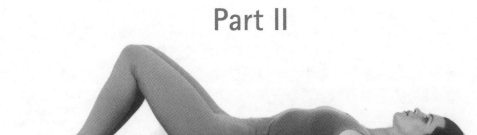

Where to start

This section provides information about what makes up our moving body. It develops the Pilates principles and introduces concepts on observation, posture and the basic anatomy of the body in a basic exercise programme that is safe for most people to do at home.

7 When is supervision required?

Return to Life was a follow-along exercise manual in which the *shapes* of the exercises were always secondary to how exercises were *done*. You were guided on how to move while you were exercising, supervising yourself. Guidance and instruction are an important part of modern Pilates (particularly if you have any injuries) because developing an acute awareness of your own body is very difficult to do by yourself. If you do have any problems it is best to attend a recognised Pilates method studio.

The instructor at a Pilates studio could be likened to an interactive 3-D mirror, helping you see which part of your body is overworking and encouraging you to connect more strongly with the most appropriate underworked muscles. When learning something new each of us responds to different ways of describing a thought or action. Everyone interprets things individually, so in this book I try to describe ideas, and repeat concepts, in slightly different ways to encompass the individual ways we learn.

Our bodies are inherently lazy. They try to do things with as little effort and thought as possible, relying on ingrained habits of movement. (In a way, it's rather like how you drive a car—you don't usually think about *how* you drive, unless you are on L-plates.) Even if you work hard, your body lets the already strong muscles work hardest. Learning how to look after your body means you need to be familiar with which muscles are tight or flexible, weak or strong; and aware of how your body feels. Being highly aware (thoughtful) of your whole body is important in order to be able to connect with and work the weaker muscles, not just the strong ones.

If you primarily use your thighs when you exercise they will become very strong. Your thighs will automatically do as much work as possible, even if you have other muscles that are better designed to make a particular movement. For example, doing a stomach crunch or curl-up is supposed to work all your stomach muscles—but how often can you feel the front of your thighs clenching and doing most of the work? Modern Pilates will help you to get all the muscles of the body working in balance.

By following the guidelines in this book, and applying the principles of the modern Pilates method to your body in a gentle way, you can improve your posture and general fitness without strain or injury. If you wish to attempt more complex work it is best to attend a reputable Pilates studio.

How to use this book

Since most of this work is done on the floor it is worthwhile buying a mat to exercise on. Lying on a hard surface is not good for you and a bed is usually too soft.

Make yourself familiar with the principles outlined in the first chapter before you start. Then turn to the guidelines following to develop a focused awareness; learn about your body by working through the journey around your body. After reading the section on body types and postural alignment, practise recognising the different postures and body types, perhaps with the help of a friend, by looking at your own and your friend's postures. This will improve your own body awareness. Get to know what muscles make you move and how you can overuse or strain different parts.

Practise the breathing, finding neutral spine and good body alignment a couple of times a day, every day for at least a week, before attempting the other exercises. In the second week add the first 2 to 4 foundation exercises, practising these a few times before adding the next 2 to 4 exercises. Steadily build on your movement ability by adding a few more exercises each week till you have completed all the basic exercises. As you become familiar with the exercises they will unwind and relax, as well as tone, the muscles.

Focused awareness

Getting to know your body from the inside out requires concentration, awareness and the ability to observe yourself impartially. The most straightforward way is for someone with a trained eye to watch you move. You can also look at yourself from the outside by using a large full-length mirror, though this can cause you to distort your posture. You can observe yourself from the inside by thinking and listening to your body and feeling with your hands which muscles are working. Another way is to have a friendly partner help (someone whom you are sure is sympathetic and who will read this book with you).

Look at your body outline in a mirror. What shape does it make? Get to know it without judging it. Are the joints big or small, loose or tight? Do you have a broad and short frame, or is it long and narrow? Do your muscles increase easily in size when you do a bit of exercise? When you have identified your basic body type, you will know what type of exercise you need to concentrate on and what you need do less of. We all are born with specific body characteristics and need to make allowances for particular genetic predispositions. Observing your body from the outside is the start of understanding it. Being familiar with the things that make up your body structure, such as bones and muscles, knowing where they are and what they do, will help considerably in focusing that understanding.

Your bones (or skeleton) are your internal support structure but they do not hold you up by themselves—muscles, tendons and ligaments connect, hold and move your body. Standing in front of a full-length mirror, have a good look at your body and identify on it the bony landmarks shown in the diagram.

Check whether the two sides of your body are in the same alignment by looking at the bony landmarks. You should see some variations in height with some of these body shapes. Everyone is a little crooked. That's what makes us recognisably ourselves.

All the movements of the body can be described quite precisely in relation to the front of the body in the standing position; see the box headed **Movement terminology**.

The Pilates Method focuses on moving with economy and grace. Connecting with, and sensing the muscles is therefore important. Becoming familiar with your body by feeling or touching it in a deliberate, thoughtful way is called palpating the muscles. Palpating your muscles will let you be aware of your muscle tone. Muscles can feel soft, firm, tight, woody, slack, springy or resilient. Using the pads of your fingers, touch the different muscles and feel under the

Movement terminology

Flexion: angle between two body parts decreases (e.g., bending the arm and bringing the hand to the shoulder)

Extension: angle between two body parts increases (e.g., straightening the leg behind the hip)

Adduction: to move towards the midline of the body (e.g., bringing the arm down to the body and inwards)

Abduction: to move away from the midline of the body (e.g., raising the leg out to the side)

External rotation: rotation of a limb outward from the body (e.g., turning the leg outward)

Internal rotation: rotation of a limb inward towards the body (e.g., pigeon toes)

Pronation: to turn the palm down; to flatten the foot

Supination: to turn the palm up; to turn up the arch of the foot

surface. This will help you identify them more specifically and increase your awareness of them.

Using the muscle diagram, begin to identify different muscles. This will help you isolate and correct muscle work. It is easiest to touch the front of the body all over but you can also feel the backs of the legs, the buttocks and some of the back as well as the shoulders, neck and head. It's not necessary to identify all the muscles; just the larger surface muscles to start with. Muscles are attached to the bony skeleton via tendons. When you are touching your body you should be able to feel the difference in texture. The tendons are the usually narrow and slightly stringy ends that attach the muscles to the bones; the muscles tend to broaden and thicken with a spongy feel in the middle.

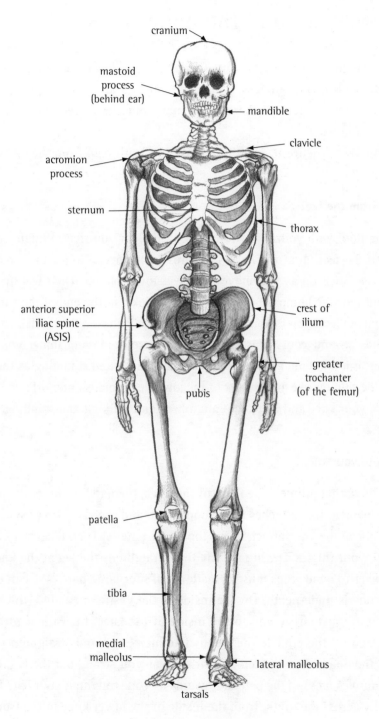

The bony landmarks of the body

8   A journey around the body

Journey around the body by looking, touching from the outside and sensing from the inside, with mental images, where the muscles are located. Try journeying around one part at a time as there are so many muscles to become familiar with, both front and back.

Starting with the front, identify the muscles with help from the diagram.

Starting from the feet

Sit on the floor with your legs stretched out, look at your feet. Wiggle your toes, then bend the feet up at the ankles towards your knees. Notice the tendons and muscles that stick up as you move your feet towards you. Then feel around the ankle bones for the bumps at either side of the ankle at the end of the shin bones. (The lateral malleolus on the outside, the medial malleolus on the inside). Then move your hands around your shins and feel the muscles moving under your hands, becoming firm and bunching as they work, softening and slimming as they relax. Identify the shin muscle at the front of the lower leg (tibialis anterior) that lifts your foot up to your knee and helps foot alignment and walking and standing.

Move up to your knees

Feel the bone that protects the front of the knee, the patella. Under the patella is a tough ligament that attaches to the upper shin and travels up to the patella. The muscles above the knee attach to the top of the patella. Then feel above the knee and up to your thighs. The big muscle that straightens the leg at the knee is the large, powerful quadriceps muscle, made up of four large parts. We can only feel three as one is underneath. On the inside is the vastus medialis, which should bulge slightly just above and to the inside of the knee, then the central rectus femoris, and on the outside the vastus lateralis. Bend and straighten your leg, and feel the quadriceps tighten and firm up as you straighten the leg. Can you see the muscles moving the patella upwards as you straighten your leg? Running diagonally across the thigh, from the inside of the lower knee to the front of the rim of the pelvis runs the sartorius muscle.

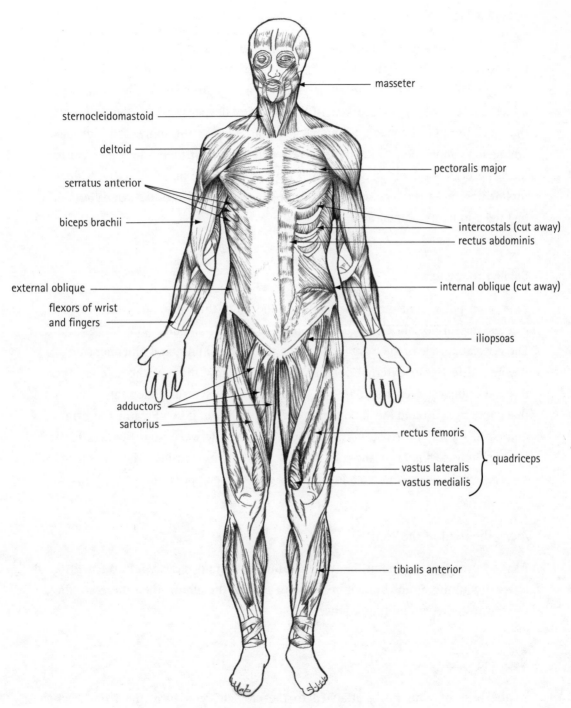

masseter

sternocleidomastoid

deltoid

pectoralis major

serratus anterior

biceps brachii

intercostals (cut away)

rectus abdominis

external oblique

internal oblique (cut away)

flexors of wrist
and fingers

iliopsoas

adductors

sartorius

rectus femoris

quadriceps

vastus lateralis

vastus medialis

tibialis anterior

Anterior muscles of the body

Going up the thigh

At the top of the leg three parts of the quadriceps attach to the front of the femur (thighbone), the fourth, the rectus femoris, attaches to the pelvis slightly to the outside of the mid-line of the groin. At the point nearest where the quadriceps attach you can often just feel one of the complex deeper muscles, the iliopsoas, that goes through the pelvis to the back and attaches to the spine. The iliopsoas and rectus femoris help to bend (flex) the leg at the hip, bringing the femur closer to the pelvis. On the inside of the upper leg lies a triangle of muscles, the adductors, which bring the legs together. If you squeeze your knees together you can feel the adductors tighten as they work.

Coming to the torso

From your pubic bone out to the hipbones and up to the bottom of your ribs you can feel the surface muscles of the abdomen, running from pubic bone to sternum. The vertical muscle in the front is called the rectus abdominis, and on either side of it you can feel your external obliques. Running below these at the side are the internal obliques; deeper still are the wraparound transversus abdominis muscles that come right around the abdomen in the deepest layer. If you breathe out firmly and narrow your waist you may feel them working. Between your ribs you have layers of muscle similar to those in the abdomen, the intercostals. The fan-shaped pectorals run upward and outward from the ribs to the upper arm.

Along the front of the arms

At the front of your arm, at the top, the anterior deltoid raises your arm; a little lower down, the biceps brachii bends your arm at the elbow, then there are the flexors of the wrist and finger muscles.

Neck and face

At the base of your neck, attached to the clavicle, you have the front neck muscle or sternocleidomastoid. The masseter muscles which control the jaw are important; if you press your teeth together you can feel these powerful muscles working in front of your ears.

Muscles from the back

Starting from your feet

Still sitting on the floor, first look at, then touch the underneath of your feet. On the soles of your feet are the plantar muscles; scrunch your toes under to feel them work. Move your toes up and down and feel the muscles on the soles of your feet. Then feel up the back of your ankle where the Achilles tendon is—this is the easiest tendon in the body to feel. Travel up your calves; when you point your foot down you can feel the two rounded bulges of the gastrocnemius working. Above that is the hollow at the back of the knee. When you bend or flex your knee the gastrocnemius (calf muscle) and the muscles of the back of the upper thigh help to create this movement and increase the hollow behind the knee. Now as you bend your leg feel these muscles at the back of your thigh—the hamstrings—which travel from below the back of the knee up to the base of the pelvis and attach to our sitting bones (the ischial tuberosities), the pointy bones one each side at the base of the pelvis. Three muscles make up your hamstring. On the inside of the leg are the semitendinosus and semimembranosus, and toward the outer side of the back of the thigh is the biceps femoris. These muscles perform two functions, bending (flexing) the leg at the knee and lifting the leg backward away from the front of the body, also called extending the leg at the hip.

Standing up

The outer or most superficial buttock muscle, the gluteus maximus, travels across the top of the back of the thigh, from the outside of the upper leg and the hip and across the back of the pelvis to the base of the spine, attaching to the sacrum in a diagonal upward sweep. This powerful muscle helps extend the leg back and also turn it outwards (externally rotate), and squeezes the bottom together. Two other gluteal muscles: at the top and to the side of the pelvic rim

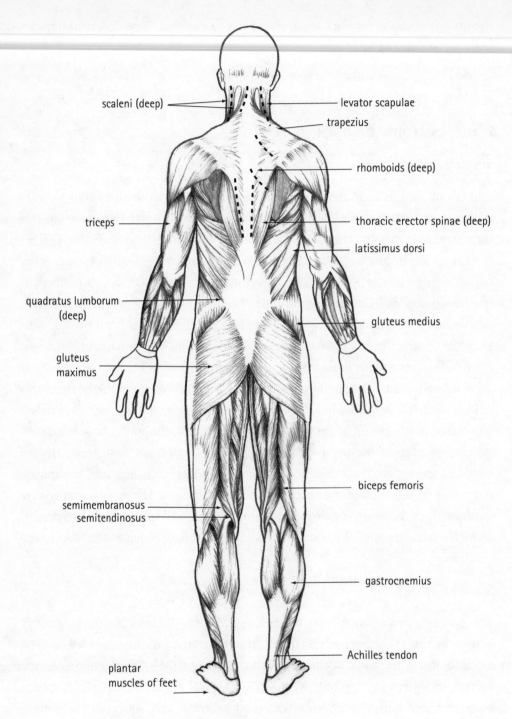

scaleni (deep)

levator scapulae

trapezius

rhomboids (deep)

triceps

thoracic erector spinae (deep)

latissimus dorsi

quadratus lumborum
(deep)

gluteus medius

gluteus
maximus

biceps femoris

semimembranosus
semitendinosus

gastrocnemius

Achilles tendon

plantar
muscles of feet

Posterior muscles of the body

you can feel the top of the gluteus medius, a muscle that goes under the gluteus maximus. This muscle also helps extend the leg and stops your body swaying too far to the side when you stand on one leg. The tensor fascia latae, directly on the side of the hip, also helps stabilise sideways sway. Many important deep posterior bottom muscles that help control the legs and pelvis can't be felt so easily; these are the deep external rotators, which primarily travel horizontally from the hip to the sacrum.

Now the torso

Touching the back of your body is quite difficult. Most people are unable to reach all of the back, as this requires very flexible shoulders and arms. On the lower back there is not much muscle bulk between pelvis and ribs. On either side there is a small deep muscle between the lower ribs and the back of the pelvis called the quadratus lumborum which you may be able to feel by pushing deeper in with your finger. The large, strong spinal muscles running straight up the sides of the vertebrae are called the erector spinae.

The sheet-like latissimus dorsi travels up from the lower back to the front of the arms via the armpits. Across the upper back and neck lies the trapezius, a diamond-shaped muscle which travels from the upper spine out to the tips of the shoulders and up the neck. It is very hard to feel the lower edge of this muscle, as it attaches into the spine at the middle of the upper back. The upper part is easy to feel. So is the upper part of the rhomboid which attaches to the inside edge of the scapula (shoulder blades) and travels diagonally to the upper spine. The rhomboids pull the shoulders together and up, and these often suffer from overwork.

Moving on to the arms

From the back of the scapula some of the shoulder muscles curve around to the side attaching into the top of the arm at the humerus. The triceps at the back of the upper arm straightens the arm. Below the triceps lie the extensors of the wrist, travelling downwards from the knob at the outside of the elbow along the back of the forearm; they also lift and straighten the fingers.

The muscles from the side

Starting from the feet

Sitting on the floor, again, you will be able to feel on either side of the foot and ankle the slender 'stirrup' muscles—the peroneus longus and peroneus brevis on the outside, and the tibialis posterior on the inside. They travel up the side of the lower leg and help stabilise the ankle; if you turn your foot over, inward and outward (pronate and supinate) you can feel them working.

The upper leg

Move to the outside of the leg. From the knob at the top of the fibula on the side of the shin there is a thin tendonous band that travels right up the outside of the upper leg to the pelvis; it is called the iliotibial band (ITB) with a muscle at the top. The tensor fascia latae, attached to the rim of the pelvis (next to the rectus femoris), moves the leg out sideways away from the centre (abducts) and stops you falling over when you stand on one leg. Just in front of the ITB, but still at the side, some parts of the vastus lateralis (a quadriceps muscle that travels up the leg) can be felt. At the side of the hip you can feel part of the gluteus medius and part of the gluteus maximus, which sweeps around the buttock and down to the upper part of the outer thigh. On the inside of your upper thigh are the adductors, muscles which also help you balance and reduce lateral sway. Try squeezing a cushion between your knees to feel these working.

Moving up to the torso

At the waist are the lateral obliques. If you bend your body sideways, and twist or turn at the waist, you can feel them work. On the outside are the sheet muscles of the external obliques, underneath them are the internal obliques. They cross diagonally at right angles, lying on the side of the waist up to the ribs. Between the ribs are the intercostal muscles: the serratus anterior runs from beneath the shoulder blade, diagonally around the ribs, a finger-shaped muscle which wraps around the ribs from under the armpit. Draw your shoulder blades down and around to feel this subtle and complex muscle work.

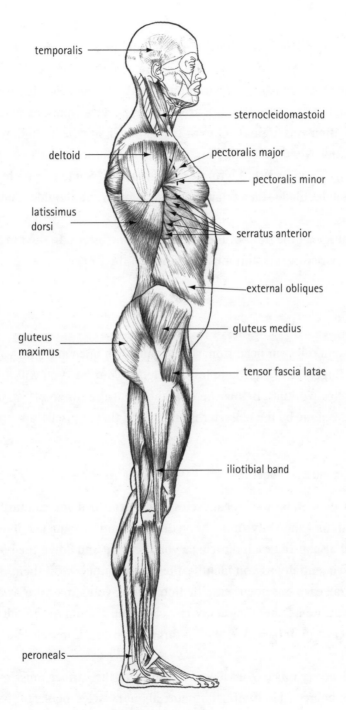

temporalis

sternocleidomastoid

deltoid

pectoralis major

pectoralis minor

latissimus dorsi

serratus anterior

external obliques

gluteus medius

gluteus maximus

tensor fascia latae

iliotibial band

peroneals

Lateral muscles of the body

Shoulders and arms

Lift one arm up and down and feel the hollow of your armpit, then the muscles at the front and back that form the hollow. Are they floppy and slack, or tight and stringy? At the back of the armpits are several muscles, including the latissimus dorsi. At the front of the armpit, the pectoral muscles across the upper chest are often very tight. On top of the shoulder sits the deltoid, which you can feel working when you lift your arm up. The other muscles supporting and moving the shoulder are the rotator cuff muscles. Some can be felt at the back of the shoulder blade—they wrap around the top of the shoulder and attach under the deltoid.

The muscle at the front of the upper arm is the biceps. In the forearm you have numerous wrist flexors and muscles that curl the fingers.

Neck and face

Lie down and roll your head from side to side, then open and shut your jaw. If you put your fingers over your temples and clench your jaw you will feel the temporalis muscles working. Below the cheekbone, at the hinge of the jaw, the same clenching is done by the masseter muscle. Both these muscles are often overtight.

Putting the muscles together

Once you are familiar with the muscles I have described you can turn this learning journey around the body into a travelling relaxation sequence by staying lying down and visualising each muscle as you focus up and down the body. Tense the muscles sequentially as you identify them and connect with them. Then let them go and relax each one down into the floor before you move your awareness to the next muscle. Remember that many muscles wrap around to the sides of the body from either front or back. We tend to forget about these muscles but they are also important.

This is a very quick overview of the some of the surface muscles of the body. (If you are interested in finding out more about muscles, books for further reading are suggested in the Bibliography.)

What happens on the surface of our bodies gives us clues about what is happening inside the body, as all the muscles attached to the bones just under the surface interact with the deeper muscles. These are the muscles which do the majority of the work involved in holding us upright—the postural, dynamic, stabilising muscles.

9 Body types and postural alignment

Body types

Our body shape and movement ability is a mixture of what we are born with (inherited) and what we use frequently (experience-modified habits). We do not just get our eye colour from our parents; we often have a similar shape and stance to our parents; sometimes we even move like one of them. You may have seen how some families echo each other's gait, mannerisms and gestures.

One of the many ways of describing body types uses a simple classification into the three main types shown in the diagram. Referring back to such a basic classification system may improve our awareness of how we move, stand and sit. Most of us, however, are mixtures of two types—for example, meso-ectomorph, meso-endomorph, and an unique mixture of strengths and weaknesses. Each body type benefits from different styles of movement and has various strengths and weaknesses that respond differently to exercise. Awareness of our basic body type helps us focus on the most useful type of exercise, and can help us understand how we function on the inside.

Body type influences posture and movement abilities, body shape, height and weight, the strength and flexibility of joint structures and the ability of muscles to work and rest. Some of us are better at short-acting, fast and strong body work, others are inherently more flexible. Some people can relax more easily. Joint laxity, muscle bulk and digestive speed all relate to body type. When you begin the exercises, target some of the movement styles that do not come naturally to your body type—do not focus only on the things that are easy.

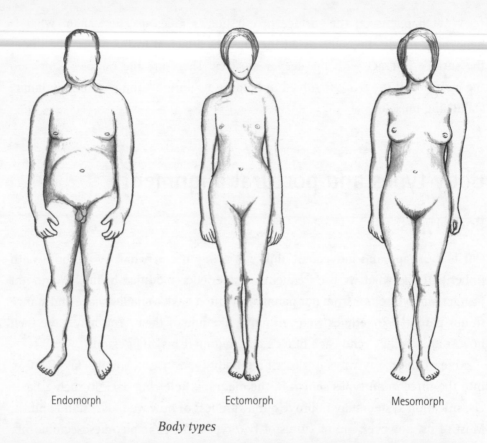

Endomorph Ectomorph Mesomorph

Body types

Body type: strengths and weaknesses

Endomorph	*Ectomorph*	*Mesomorph*
good cardiovascular system	poor cardiovascular system	excellent circulation
eats a little, stores it all	eats a lot, still thin	eats well, moderate weight
medium heart rate	high heart rate	low heart rate
moderate joints	very floppy joints	strong joints
muscles hide under fat	could never be body-builder	grows muscle easily
broad	tall, slender, long legs	shorter, chunky

Good:	Good:	Good:
excellent relaxation	quick reaction time	excellent strength
good muscle endurance	speed for short duration	excellent muscle
	elasticity	endurance
Poor:	**Poor:**	**Poor:**
weight control	strength	flexibility
fast movement	muscle endurance	extremes fast, slow
	relaxation	

Postural alignment

Posture is how we hold our body, how our limbs, head and torso are aligned in space. Different postures mean that we hold and use our inner or deeper muscles in particular ways. Being familiar with our own postural alignment helps us be aware of what inner muscles are overworking, underworking or fixed. Current thinking in Pilates brings together the ideas of moving and holding (supporting) at the same time, sometimes called dynamic stabilisation.

Various postural models have been developed over the last few decades. Kendall, for example, devised and labelled a series of basic body postures, including ideal, sway, kypho/lordosis and flat. Each postural variation commonly overuses different groups of muscles which hold that particular posture. Thus, having an awareness of these postures can help our understanding of what internal muscles may be either tight or underworked.

Asymmetry and scoliosis

Much fuss is made about being asymmetrical—but being asymmetrical is *not* an illness. Most people are asymmetrical. From the length of the feet to the formation of the teeth, the two sides of the body are slightly different. It is largely because we are either right- or left-handed—the body adapts and muscles

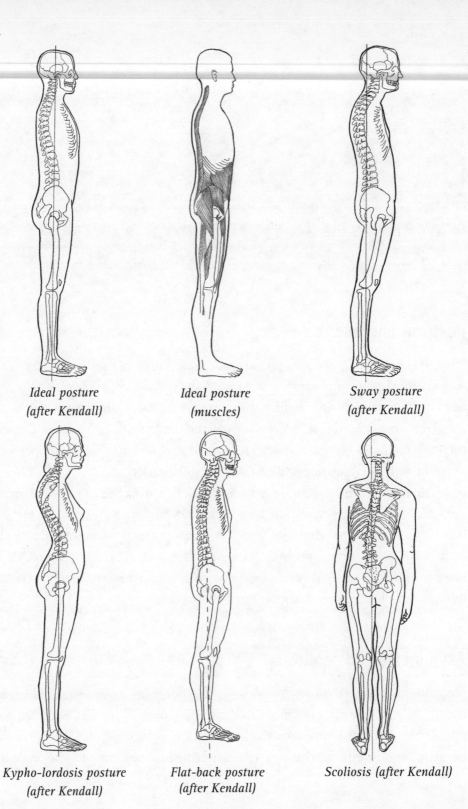

Ideal posture
(after Kendall)

Ideal posture
(muscles)

Sway posture
(after Kendall)

Kypho-lordosis posture
(after Kendall)

Flat-back posture
(after Kendall)

Scoliosis (after Kendall)

strengthen asymmetrically in response. That is called a functional scoliosis, and is completely natural and normal. A very small percentage of the population are structurally so asymmetrical that they have uneven movements and noticeably uneven stance. Like many other things, a little bit of scoliosis is okay and nothing to worry about. There are two basic types of scoliosis: C, where the back traces a large C shape in one curve, and S, where the back makes a gentle S shape with two curves. Where asymmetry does not allow you to function properly, or is out of balance, poorly compensated and causing discomfort, you need to be looked at by a medical specialist or a good manual therapist, and attend a Pilates studio run by an especially skilled practitioner.

Recognising your general body shape and posture can be quite difficult. You need mirrors set at an angle to see your spine and to look at yourself side on. Preferably with an impartial partner, observe yourself from all directions to identify your basic posture. People often have strong beliefs about how to stand or sit 'properly'. We also need to be aware of how we stand or sit when we are tired, tense stressed or relaxed. When you do relax be aware of what happens to your body. Also what muscles are still working when we lie down to rest—some muscles just don't want to turn off.

Posture and emotions

Posture is affected by how you feel, by your emotional state. What does your body do when you concentrate for long periods or experience a strong emotion such as happiness, sadness or anger. Not only will you hold your body differently but sustaining a particular emotion for a long period of time, causes your body to retain that posture (muscle memory). So being aware of our bodies is not just being aware of the shapes that we make with our muscles, bones and joints, it is being aware of how we feel. Our muscles can reflect our emotional state. Think of how you hold yourself in different situations—when you are 'on show', for example, making an effort to impress. Do you have a different posture for everyday—a working posture? What happens to your posture when you are relaxed? In the 1970s Phil Latey developed the idea of postural layers.

We all have a public posture, a good or alert posture which we use when meeting new people, or at a work conference. We also have a relaxed (slumped) posture, used when we unwind after a difficult day at work, a comfortable at-home posture for when no one is looking. We do not just dress differently for different situations, our posture changes to match the situation.

Our socially alert posture or 'image' posture is often tense. How many of us during our teenage years were told by our parents to 'stand up straight and pull your shoulders back'? Even as adults we may feel that our parents knew what they were talking about and occasionally unconsciously oblige. How you sit at a desk is reminiscent of school—did you hunch over your desk? How fast did you grow, how large and how early did your breasts grow, did you have acne? These things all affect our postural alignment. Our body habits generally become ingrained quite early, with fixed postural layers developing during our adolescence and early twenties.

These primarily upright postures are strongly affected by gravity. To retrain your body to a better upright posture you will need to give the supporting muscles a chance to let go by changing their response to gravity. Sometimes muscles still work even though they don't need to hold us upright. What happens when we lie down? What muscles are still working when we rest? Some postural muscles can become fixed in a shortened working state. Awareness of this (residual) posture lets us know which much deeper and chronically overworked muscles are still working when we are at rest. They are often holding on to the very deep restrictions that are inhibiting our enjoyment of life.

Starting to improve your awareness, by lying down in a supported rest position (see pp. 71–2), lets you focus on your inner postural muscles, and reduces the effect of gravity on your body. The supported rest position is a very good

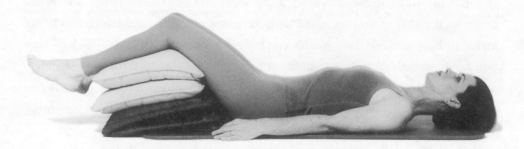

Supported rest position

place to start to exercise and begin to improve your postural alignment. You want to unwind the tight bits as well as stretch and strengthen the weak parts of your body.

10 How to connect with your body

Our ability to see and touch our bodies, combined with knowledge of which muscles do what, allows us to connect the outside (surface) with the inside (internal workings).

We can observe shape and posture. We know that different postures can make certain muscles overwork. Be aware of the different levels of posture, from alert image to relaxed slump to the underlying residual. The deepest muscles involved in poor postural habits are much harder to connect with than surface muscles. Overused deep postural muscles send messages to the brain when they are working too hard, but we often ignore them until they are aching with strain and refuse to do more. They may turn numb and rigid. When you cannot hear your body telling you that it needs a break, something is bound to snap, strain or go on strike.

Apply the foundation principle of the Pilates method by focusing awareness on yourself. By directing your mind to concentrate and feel what your body is doing, you will be able to exercise the precise muscles you want to use, which will give you the opportunity to internally redirect overworked muscles.

Pathways to the mind

Joe Pilates always said, 'It is the mind that controls the body.'

The paradox here is that in the Pilates method we put huge effort into understanding and improving our awareness so that we can acquire good body habits and move with grace and efficiency *without having to think about it* (as Friedman and Eisen noted).

The mind relates to the body via the nervous system. It controls both involuntary and voluntary activity. The nervous system is made up of the central nervous system (CNS) and the peripheral nervous system (PNS). The CNS is made up of the brain and spinal cord and processes the information that our body and its senses send to it. It can be likened to the mainframe computer in a network. The peripheral nervous system consists of all the nerves throughout the rest of the body and can be subdivided into the autonomic (involuntary) nervous system (which is, in turn, further subdivided into the sympathetic and parasympathetic nervous systems and controls aspects of the body's background functions), the somatic (voluntary) and sensory nerves.

We can think of the autonomic system as our own personal autopilot. If you are stressed your body's systems speed up and you become alert, the body going into fight or flight mode ready to protect you (sympathetic nervous system); when the emergency is over, you begin to relax and calm down and your body restarts its peaceful metabolism (parasympathetic nervous system).

The somatic nerves connected to your muscles and skin (body voluntary system) tell the brain when your body is hot or cold, what you are touching, whether a muscle is stretched, overstretched or tired and what position your joints are at—it tells you what position in space your body is maintaining.

There are many automatic (unconscious) response patterns or reflexes that safeguard the body, such as the postural righting reflex and the stretch reflex, which is a reflexive contraction of muscle immediately after it has been stretched, a protective mechanism that can prevent the overextension of a joint. The golgi tendon reflex protects the muscles and their tendons: if there is such extreme pull or stretch on a muscle that the tendon is about to be pulled off the bone, the muscle lets go completely and relaxes like jelly. This response is unfortunately so last-minute that sometimes the tendon tears away as the body cannot react to the reflex quickly enough. This means we need to be careful when overriding our reflexes.

The reflex of reciprocal inhibition also acts to prevent muscle injury; when one muscle shortens quickly, the opposing muscle lengthens and relaxes and is reciprocally inhibited or stopped from working. This reflex can be used along with the stretch reflex to assist in increasing stretch. Active resisted-movement exercises can be designed to work a muscle in its lengthened state, so that it relaxes and lengthens further.

Over time some reflex actions can be conditioned or altered so as to improve

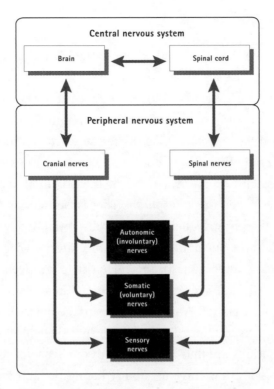

Division of the nervous system (after Hinkle)

and simplify movement habits. We can use this knowledge of reflexes and complex nervous system behaviour to improve the qualityof our exercise and avoid injury.

Sometimes we become so disconnected from our bodies that we lose sensation, we feel numb. It is a bit like a radio turned down very low—we can hear or feel some noise but can't make out what's being said. This often happens when we are injured, and especially when we are tired, stressed or shocked. We can protect and balance our bodies much better when we can feel and sense them more clearly and strongly.

So, lying down, be aware, concentrate on what muscles are still working. Move your focus around your body to turn up the volume on what it is telling you. Be aware if an area is hard to connect to. Are the fronts of the hips tight? What are your neck and shoulders doing? Is your spine arched or resting on the floor? Is there any pain or discomfort or tension or numbness?

Sensing sensation

You connect with your body by thinking and listening to the feelings (messages) it sends to your brain. We are all aware of the five senses of sight, hearing, smell, taste and touch, but we have other senses too. A sense of 'bodilyness', that arises from internal movement in our muscles and the relative position of body parts, is sometimes called the muscle or kinaesthetic sense. It is also linked to feelings of pain and temperature. A second bodily sense relates to external space, place or movement possibilities, an awareness of the potential space the body can occupy (sometimes called the kinesphere). That is, sensations from our muscles tell us that we have a physical 'beingness', a substantial bodilyness in the world. The sense of activity in our brain and the more internal, deep visceral muscle sensations are equally important, for they give rise to 'gut feelings' and the more intense emotions. All these senses link and interact in an emotive feedback loop to our brain. So the sensations we feel in our surface muscles, skin and internal organs react with the sensations felt by our deeper skeletal muscles.

Muscular sensations are thus a huge part of our sense of self. By quietening the big strong muscles that move us, and reducing the activity of our postural muscles, we can connect with the subtler feelings that come from all the muscles and joints, including the deeper postural and visceral muscles that help with bodily functions such as digestion and breathing. Our deep postural and inner muscles can unwind and be retrained as we learn to use the variable volume control in our ability to sense sensations.

11 Breathing

Breathing is the first thing to learn.

> . . . To breathe correctly you must completely exhale and inhale, always trying very hard to 'squeeze' every atom of impure air from your lungs in much the same manner that you would wring every drop of water from a wet cloth . . . the lungs will automatically completely

refill themselves with fresh air. This in turn supplies the bloodstream with vitally necessary life-giving oxygen. Also the complete exhalation and inhalation of air stimulates all the muscles into greater activity . . . Lazy breathing converts the lungs, figuratively speaking, into a cemetery for the deposition of diseased, dying and dead germs . . . (Return to Life, p. 13).

What is breathing or respiration?

Breathing is the means by which the body replenishes itself with fresh gases, acquiring oxygen, and eliminates waste gases (among them carbon dioxide), using the blood as a carrier to and from the lungs, where the exchange takes place. Oxygen is the primary key to unlocking the body's energy—it is the fuel for aerobic activity.

Breathing is the first act of life, and the last

There is no single correct way to breathe, but there are many inappropriate ways (bad habits). Getting to know how breathing works will help you find the most efficient way.

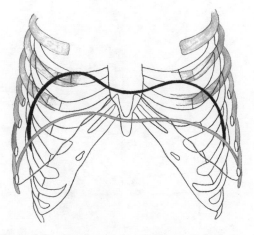

Portion of the diaphragm in maximum inhalation (grey) and exhalation (black)

In quiet breathing the effort phase occurs only during inhalation—when you breathe in. Muscular effort is required to enlarge the thoracic cavity and lower intra-thoracic pressure sufficiently to move gases into the lungs. This quiet breathing is performed by the muscles of the thorax. The abdomen expands passively in response to the change in volume in the chest. Exhalation (breathing out) results from the elastic recoil of the lungs upon relaxation of the muscles of inhalation. The muscles of exhalation become active, however, when the demands of breathing are increased. The abdominal muscles then actively help exhalation, minimising effort in the upper chest and assisting the diaphragm.

The diaphragm is the prime muscle of breathing. It is a big complex muscle like an upturned elastic bowl in a double dome shape. It draws down and becomes shallow and broad on inhalation, and curves upwards, with the rim of the bowl narrowing, on exhalation. It is helped by the muscles of the ribcage, mid and upper back muscles, the abdominal muscles, neck and shoulder muscles.

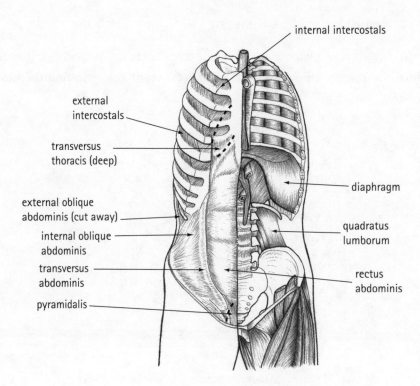

The muscles of the torso

Almost all the muscles involved in breathing also have a *postural* function. Thus breathing and posture do have a strong connection, as Pilates said in *Your Health*.

When you breathe the diaphragm moves up and down and affects the contents and size of the abdomen, unless there are restrictions on this motion. Very weak, protruding abdominal muscles reduce the ability to breathe out deeply when we put extra demands on the body. Non-responsive tight abdominals restrict the flow of movement in the diaphragm and tense up the back, limiting the volume of the chest and reducing maximum lung capacity.

The most efficient way to breathe is to use your body without restriction or tightness or excessive effort. A free-flowing exchange of air, with a gentle rhythm through the body, is like the rhythm section in a band, underpinning all the bodily systems.

Breathing is one of a number of internal automatic activities of the body, along with pumping blood through the circulatory system, digesting food and so on. Breathing is also the one involuntary function or internal activity that is both unconscious and conscious. Breathing's high dependence on large muscle activity, and the sensations we feel in those muscles, provides us with the ability to connect with and influence the process of breathing. Through being aware of and focusing on breathing, we can draw our attention inwards and engage our deeper postural muscles.

Breathing is vital for life and is readily affected by physical effort, mental effort and emotion. How often do we hold our breath when we study, lift something heavy or restrain our anger? Do you hold your tongue? How do you hold still? Let go when crying? Our breathing is intimately linked and resonates with our ability to express or repress emotions.

Types of breathing

Always remember the words of Uncle Joe: 'Even if you follow no other instructions, learn to breathe correctly'.

Getting to know and be aware of breathing patterns is vital to modern Pilates and to helping change ingrained and inappropriate body habits. Take time to observe how you breathe in different situations. Do you primarily breathe with just your neck and shoulders, or do you only flare out the lower ribs and hollow

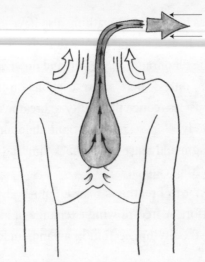

Siphon breathing—the movement direction is upward and narrowing

the stomach? Do you bulge your abdomen and hold your ribs still? Do you do a mixture of these things?

We can divide breathing into three basic actions, referred to as 'siphon', 'bellows', and 'piston'.

Siphon

In the siphon action the neck and throat tighten, trying to suck air in, and the shoulders elevate. The abdominal muscles remain soft or disconnected. The chest lifts forward with the neck and upper thorax tense, and the upper body is elevated with the help of the mid and upper back and shoulder muscles. Imagine sucking thick syrup through a straw. This type of breathing overuses the upper accessory muscles of inspiration, the scaleni plus the trapezius, levator scapula and serratus posterior superior (see pages 36 and 39). The ribs may stay narrowed, though the sternum lifts. The waist appears to shrink flaccidly on inhalation but this is due to the elevation of the ribs and lifting of the upper chest.

Bellows

In the bellows action the ribs flare apart and upwards (like the two handles on a bucket) as we breathe in, with the intercostal muscles between the ribs working together with the diaphragm, which broadens out as its central tendon is lowered.

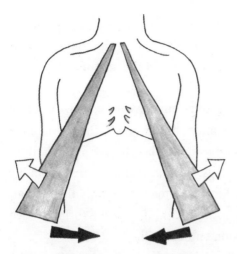 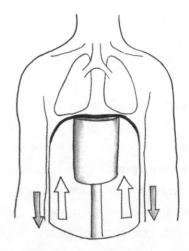

Bellows breathing—the movement direc-
tion is sideward and outward

Piston breathing—the movement flows
downward and slightly outward
into the whole abdominal cavity

There is minimal abdominal movement in bellows breathing. The abdominal muscles are relatively still and act to support the front of the body, in isometric contraction. When the downward movement of the contents of the abdomen is resisted, there is more elevation and expansion of the upper rib cage on the inhalation in bellows breathing than in siphon breathing.

Piston

In the piston action, the lowering work of the diaphragm on the inhalation is assisted by the intercostals moving more outwards and sideways than upward. With resilient abdominals, this movement gently presses the contents of the abdomen toward the pelvic floor, expanding out and down the body. The psoas muscles probably work to anchor the effort of the diaphragm. Support for this action comes from the eccentric work of the transversus abdominis and obliques.

On the exhalation the pelvic floor muscles draw up the lower abdomen with the lower obliques. The shortening of the transversus abdominis brings the fibres of the two diagonally opposed obliques closer together in a scissor-like action. The obliques respond by working concentrically on the exhalation (but eccentrically on the inhalation when the transversus abdominis lengthens). The rectus abdominis assists by shortening slightly, balancing the action of the tranversus on the lumbar spine and reducing lordosis. The pyramidalis muscle tightens the lowest part of the abdominal wall to support this action.

We need to use all three ways of breathing at times but for various reasons often end up relying only on one main way. Siphon breathing is the form most commonly overused, where the shoulders and upper ribs lift, the neck tightens and the throat sucks the air into the upper lungs. It is particularly stressful on the body and commonly seen in people with asthma, who tend to fill only the top part of the lungs and don't properly exhale. Bellows breathing was the form focused on in more traditional Pilates, with the abdomen held still.

The form least often used correctly is piston breathing, which is often misinterpreted as belly-bulging and for this reason avoided. I have most fully described the muscular action of piston breathing, as it has been ignored in traditional Pilates. A mixture of piston and bellows breathing is most appropriate for efficient breathing in everyday life. In modern Pilates this combination, called alert torso breathing, is encouraged with the muscle actions on exhalation exaggerated to encourage abdominal muscle work, pelvic floor function and good postural alignment. Inhaling through the nose and exhaling through the mouth, with softly parted lips helps to reduce tension in the jaw, neck and throat.

The fact that breathing can be altered by changes in position, emotional state, activity level, disease, and even tight garments, means that re-learning breathing can be a very slow process. Since many of our breathing muscles perform vital roles in assisting good postural alignment and support, working with the muscles of breathing via improving posture can assist the retraining of breathing, and vice versa. Practising modern Pilates will encourage the naturally efficient patterns to reassert themselves gradually over the long term.

In some circumstances accessory muscles come to be used as primary breathing muscles. This can happen as a result of disease (such as asthma, polio, emphysema) or due to learned inappropriate patterns of movement.

Modern Pilates uses breathing to:

- Promote abdominal strength and reduce tension in the upper body;

- Connect the pelvic floor and lower abdominals with the movement of the diaphragm;

- Improve posture and sensory awareness of the body;

- Resist the urge to hold the breath on exertion and when concentrating;

- Help with co-ordination and increase oxygen uptake.

This contrasts with the traditional Pilates method, which promotes extremely deep and full breathing, working on both the exhalation and inhalation, (and occasionally forced percussive breathing) with the abdomen held in strongly at all times. This tended to put pressure into the lower back and encouraged bracing of the abdomen. This is really appropriate only for elite athletes or the very fit on occasions of extreme exertion.

Breathing and rhythm

The rhythm of your breathing changes depending on the demands placed on your body. Some breaths may be long and full, others short and shallow. The important thing is that the exhalation is not rushed. In modern Pilates method much of the exertive work of an exercise is on the exhalation, thus you must be capable of providing enough time on your out-breath to complete the exercise's action. Lengthening the time of the breath cycle also has a calming effect.

The pause at the end of the exhalation also signals to your nervous system that it is time for the next oxygen intake. If the pause is complete, the ensuing breath-in feels effortless and full, as it has been triggered by the body's natural physiological demands.

The alert torso breathing used in modern Pilates method combines diaphragmatic breathing with an awareness of breathing into the back and down into the pelvic floor, and avoids unconscious fast exhalation.

Practise variations on breathing

Practise different types of breathing—the type taught in the original Pilates method and to the present day form. Try the vigorous full breathing of traditional Pilates—lifting your ribs up and out on the inhalation, compressing the ribs and strongly shortening your abdominals to exhale while holding the abdomen flat. Attempt strong fast breathing with minimal or no obvious movement. Then try inhaling on effort and exhaling on effort, noticing how all these variations make you feel.

In the next two exercises we will practise the different types of breathing so you become familiar with them. We all tend to use one type as our main way of breathing. Work out which breathing method you primarily use and practise the method you use less frequently.

Coordinating the use of breath to find the deep abdominals

The beauty of piston breathing is that the expansion of the abdomen allows for a good sensation and connection to the lower abdomen through using our transversus abdominis, obliques, pyramidalis muscles and the pelvic floor. The action of piston breathing gives you something to narrow—it is very hard to connect with something that is still. Exaggerating the movement initially can help connect with this often numb area—but at the same time you do not want to push out or bulge the abdomen, or press down into the pelvic floor too much, as this may overarch the back. Think of expanding into the lower back as much as into the front of the abdomen and the pelvic bowl.

BREATHING WITH A BOOK

Aim:

To connect with the action of piston breathing. It should not be confused with belly-bulging, which occurs when you use intra-abdominal pressure rather than proper abdominal work.

To start, lie down on your back, with your knees bent up, feet hip width apart on the floor and arms comfortably by your side (the constructive rest position). To

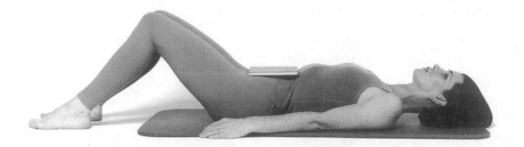

more fully relax the body, you can practise these exercises with your legs supported by pillows or resting on a chair. See pp. 71–2 for a fuller description of what is called the 'supported rest' position. Rest a small book on your lower abdomen (between your hip bones and just above your pubic bone).

Inhale through your nose, allow your breath to expand down to your lower abdomen and into your pelvic floor, letting the book rise. As you exhale, with softly parted lips, draw the lower abdomen in toward the floor, and up toward your navel, narrowing the flesh across the space between your hip bones and making the book sink downward, at the same time narrowing and drawing up your lower abdomen and lengthening your waist.

Repeat 8 times.

Visualisation:

You are zipping up a tight pair of trousers as you breathe out.

Points of caution:

Take care not to over-bulge or pop up the front of the abdomen, ensure you expand the waist sideways and down as you inhale.

BREATHING WITH A STRAP

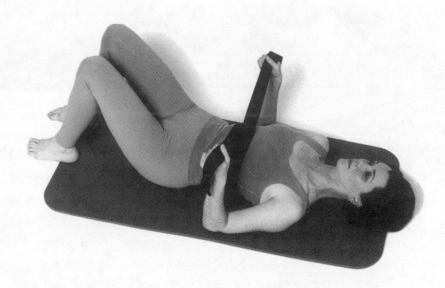

Aim:

To improve the sideways movement in the lower ribs in bellows breathing.

Lie down on your back with knees bent and feet flat on the floor. Wrap a scarf or broad belt around your lower ribs, then cross the ends above your ribs. With your arms by your sides, elbows bent, hold the ends of the scarf gently in your hands.

Inhale, letting the ribs flare and expand into the back and side of the body. Feel the scarf becoming taut around your body. Allow your hands to move towards each other slightly as the circumference of the ribs enlarges and the amount of scarf around your body lengthens. Exhale and gently draw the scarf tighter by pulling on the ends by slightly parting the hands, feeling the ribs soften down and narrow.

Repeat 8 times.

Visualisation:

Your ribs expand like the action of an accordion.

Points of caution:

Take care not to pull the ribs up towards to the base of the throat, and tense the neck.

BREATHING CONNECTED TO YOUR CENTRE—ALERT TORSO BREATHING

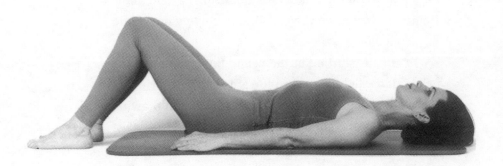

When you are comfortable with the first two exercises, practise this exercise.

Aim:

To put both types of breathing together without over-breathing.

To start, lie down on your back with your knees bent, feet on the floor hip-width apart. Gently rest your hands on your abdomen, with fingers spread out between the lower ribs to the crests of the pelvis.

Begin to inhale, first sideways into the ribs then downward into the abdomen, which expands out and down towards the pelvic floor. Pause momentarily.

To start the exhalation, push out the air, from the pelvic floor upward, by drawing in the abdomen from the pubic bone upward. Continue to exhale by narrowing your waist and softening the ribs downward.

When you are inhaling, it should feel as if you are letting the air in by drawing the ribs apart, gently filling the lungs as they expand down into the space left by the lower ribs as the diaphragm flattens and broadens. As the diaphragm flattens it pushes the contents of the abdomen downward and outward. The abdominal muscles accommodate this expansion of the viscera by expanding outward at the waist and rising upward in the front of the pelvic bowl, very slightly bulging down into the pelvic floor.

To exhale, starting at the pelvic floor you draw the pelvic floor slightly upward toward the waist, bringing the lower abdomen in and up, with a feeling of drawing up the line of the top of the pubis. Narrowing the waist softens the ribs downwards and allows the diaphragm to narrow in circumference and increase the height of its dome shape. The contents of the abdominal cavity move up slightly, into the space left by the elevation of the middle of the diaphragm.

Repeat 8 times.

Visualisation:

Imagine that a wave of breath is like a wave breaking on a beach at low tide, with the swell building out through the ribs on the inhalation and sliding up the beach, down to the pelvic floor. As you exhale the wave slides back down the beach into the sea.

Points of caution:

Take care not hold your abdomen in all the time; imagine your breath massaging your stomach.

Everything inside your body, apart from the bones, is extremely slippery, so gentle and subtle feelings of flow are normal and desirable.

Thus breathing with the middle and lower parts of the body to create a gentle wave through the body which affects the whole torso, creates internal body awareness, improves alignment and helps you find and use your centre.

This exercise connects with the exercises that find the centre and the neutral spine. Once you are comfortable with it, replace this breathing exercise with breathing in the neutral spine, which is described on page 67.

12 Introducing the modern centre

In his original book, *Your Health*, Joe Pilates writes of the link between correct breathing and natural posture, the connection which became in his teaching practice the powerhouse or initiator and centre of effort. It was also clearly outlined by Freidman and Eisen. The centre itself lay between the base of the ribs and the top of the pelvis. This area was much too high and restricted by comparison with the modern centre, missing the connection with the lower abdominals and ignoring the pelvic floor.

The modern centre is seen as the area from the diaphragm to the pelvic floor, encompassing the whole of the pelvic function and enclosing all of the viscera. The abdominal muscles surround and support the lower torso and connect the strong bony pelvis to the ribs, helping to stabilise the spine. Working from the modern centre is sometimes called 'core stabilisation'.

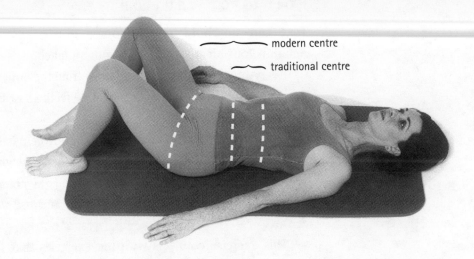

modern centre
traditional centre

It is important to really understand the abdominal muscles, because they are critically important to the whole body. This group of muscles that work together to support, hold and move the body in a complex way are often misunderstood and underused.

The four important abdominal muscles, starting from the deepest (and hardest to find), are the transversus abdominis, the internal oblique, the external oblique and the rectus abdominis, the outermost. Together they form a 'corset' from the pubic bone to the ribs, and wrap around the body to the spine at their deepest. At the front they balance the strength of the spine. They work together to contain and support the viscera, to stabilise the spine and to bend and twist the body. In exercise the rectus abdominis is the easiest to activate but it is only really useful when it is controlled by the obliques and transversus abdominis. Only when you are breathing correctly can you activate the lateral and deeper abdominal muscles correctly; the abdomen can only function well when this occurs.

Anatomy review: the abdominal muscles

The transversus abdominis forms the deepest layer. It fans out horizontally around the body from the spine at the back of the waist, joining the vertical rectus abdominis muscle at the front of the body. It spreads between the lower ribs and the pubic bone like two large hands spanning the waist. It narrows the waist, slightly extends the lower back and flattens the stomach. It also interconnects with the diaphragm.

The internal oblique, the second deepest layer, is found on both sides of the body wrapping around to the front. It travels from the crest of the pelvis and the lower fold of the groin in a diagonal pathway up and in toward the ribs, and connects with the vertical rectus abdominis. It helps bend and spirally twist the torso and also flattens the stomach.

The external oblique, the outermost side muscle, lies on top of the internal oblique on both sides of the body and goes around to the front. It travels from the lower ribs in a diagonal pathway down to the crest of the pelvis and the lower fold of the groin, and also connects with the rectus abdominis. The external oblique helps with side bending, twisting and rotation of the torso, and narrowing of the waist. It also assists in flexing the thorax, and usually interdigitates with the latissimus dorsi and serratus anterior.

The oblique muscles work synergistically (together) in rotation of the trunk. For example, right rotation of the trunk is assisted by contraction of the right internal oblique, while the left external oblique contracts eccentrically to lengthen the space between the ribs and pelvis.

The rectus abdominis, the vertical central abdominal muscle, travels in two

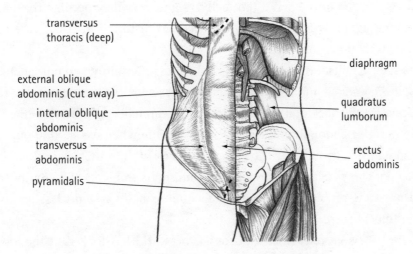

Abdominal muscles anatomy drawing

parallel bands between the pubis and the lower edge of the sternum and ribs. When highly developed it creates the 'six-pack'. It is the easiest muscle to work and is often overused, destroying its balance with the other abdominal muscles. It works to bend the body toward the pelvis, tilts the pelvis up so that the pubic bone moves toward the ribs, and assists the other abdominals to support the abdomen.

As well as the four big abdominal muscles, there is a small muscle attached to the pubic bone that tightens the mid-line join of the abdominals. The pyramidalis muscle comes up to an important line across the abdomen halfway between the belly button and the pubic bone. It works with the pelvic floor to form the very lowest part of our breathing movement.

At the back of the body other muscles of the spine and lower back, including the erector spinae group and quadratus lumborum, help support the spine. In particular, the deep multifidus (at the lumbo-sacral region) plays a subtle but vital role, via eccentric action in conjunction with the abdominals.

The iliopsoas muscles, (iliacas, psoas major and psoas minor) connecting the spine, pelvis and legs are also important muscles.

So, many muscles work, support and control the centre of the body in a complex relationship. When the big strong outer muscles are overworked they restrict the inner postural muscles from working properly. Sometimes the abdominal muscles get so little use they become lax and the viscera start flopping outward over the rim of the pelvis (pot belly); sometimes they become fixed and shortened, and again overused. The spine becomes distorted in either case and back problems may become chronic.

Pilates said, 'Civilisation impairs physical fitness'. Certainly manual labour is becoming less common, and modern living involves a lot of sitting down. We rest our spine against the back of a seat at work, in the car, relaxing in front of the TV, at a computer. Our abdominal muscles tend to be idle when we sit, and our hip flexors and hamstrings tighten. The viscera press down into the pelvic floor and the pelvic floor can weaken and stretch contributing to problems of incontinence, piles and prostrate problems. We use our locomotor body systems less and our hands and fingers more.

From the 1970s various research around the world has looked at the lower torso, as poor muscle tone here can cause so many problems, particularly in the back. This is an area of vulnerability that the Pilates method has been addressing for many decades. In the early 1990s physiotherapists noticed that working from the centre and using the principles of the Pilates method helped reduce and resolve lower back problems. Further research then began on the role of the centre in 'core stabilisation' and the reduction of spinal problems. As one physiotherapist wrote in the mid-1990s, 'Is science catching up with Pilates?', when research confirmed that the deep abdominals and spinal muscles (the centre) need to work together to support the spine. Using just the superficial back muscles was not enough.

Modern Pilates method goes much further. It does not just try to brace the spine using the deep wrap-around muscles of the abdomen. Correct centring lengthens as it strengthens and supports the torso, with all the muscles of the trunk, including the abdominal region, working together to protect the back and creating a spacious resilient neutral alignment of the whole body. Modern Pilates aims to get the whole centre working in conjunction with the limbs, integrating all of the complex spiral movements.

13 Finding postural alignment

The neutral spine

Pilates thought the spine should be straight like a plumb line (*Return to Life*) and that flattening it down to the mat helped improve its ability to retain flexibility and keep an upright posture even in old age. But this is not comfortable nor natural—if we tried to always keep a flat back we would be constantly gripping our buttocks, tucking the pelvis back, locking the iliacus in mid-range and holding the psoas tight right up through the thoracic junction. Our anatomical knowledge has improved since then, and from the early 1980s some Pilates instructors have been working in a much more relaxed natural and ergonomic position.

The early Pilates instructor Eve Gentry coined the term 'neutral spine' to refer to the most appropriate position to exercise in. At the same time some English instructors, such as Dreas Reyneke, began to move away from the traditional flattened spine and work in a natural spinal alignment. I found that working in a natural alignment when my body was changing from that of dancer to a child-bearing body, was particularly important.

Neutral or natural spinal alignment is that position which places minimal stress on the spine, where the bones are in alignment so that there is balanced muscle effort following the spine's natural forward and backward curves. Neutral spine is unique to each individual and is related to the mature shape of the vertebrae which give it its gentle curves. In neutral spine the pillows (discs) between the vertebrae are not squashed or pinched out of shape. Curves are much more resilient than a straight line, and the spine's natural forward and backward curves help absorb impact.

To find and sustain neutral spine we must engage our abdominals. Exercising in a neutral spine position protects the spine from injury, recruits the abdominal muscles to work properly and improves posture. Linking all this with breathing and coordination is an essential of modern Pilates.

Every individual's comfortable body alignment is unique. It is a combination of your bony structure, surrounding soft tissue and how you use it—that is structure and function combined. How your body lines up is controlled by the muscles and is related to the shapes of your bones. We want to align our bones and joints to cause as little stress to our bodies as possible and be in dynamic balance.

How to find neutral spine

Imprinting exercises

Eve Gentry's imprinting—letting the bones of the spine relax into the mat as though leaving an imprint in the sand—is a good way of becoming aware of spinal alignment when lying on your back. More importantly, it helps initiate the connection with the centre without your back being distorted and compressed or your pelvis tucked under.

We want to support the body in its most comfortable spinal-aligned position; we can find neutral spine most easily by taking away some of the effects of gravity in the supported rest position.

Eve Gentry developed imprinting exercises in the side lie position as well as in the supine (on your back) position, but imprinting only works effectively when you lie on your back. Since the impression of the spine is made downward, in the side lie position pressing downward increases distortion in the spinal alignment. Lateral work is discussed later in this chapter. Similarly, imprinting the neck in both supine and side lie positions can easily cause misalignment, over-compressing the front of the discs, and should only be done under supervision.

IMPRINTING

Aim:

For awareness and connecting breath and centring. This also helps with preparing to move. Done in supine position only.

This exercise is very much like the final breathing exercise, except that the focus has moved to awareness of spinal alignment. I will describe it in two parts.

Mid-and lower back

To start, lie in either rest position described on page 71–2, with the lower back relaxed on the mat.

If your lower back does not rest gently on the floor (there is a space between your back and the mat), bend one knee up to your chest, then the other knee, and gently circle both legs by holding the knees with the hands. This massages and relaxes the lower back. Return to your original position.

Inhale, being aware of the weight of the body. As you exhale draw the abdomen in and feel the spine sink down toward the floor as though leaving an imprint of your back in sand.

Repeat 8 to 10 times.

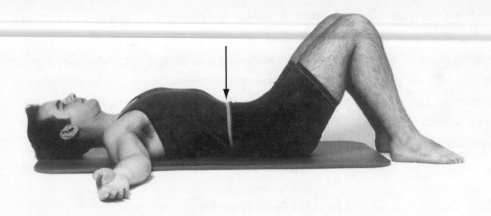

Points of caution:

Take care not to press your back over-firmly into the mat or tilt the pelvis. Maintain your alignment as it is rather than distort your posture.

Upper spine and neck

The chest (upper back) tends to sink down into the mat with its own weight but the neck has a natural curve up off the mat. If your upper spine curves forward too much you will have trouble relaxing your head into the mat and your neck will curve too much. If this is happening, place a small pillow under your head. Gently lengthen your head away from your shoulders and sink it into the mat. Think of your ears getting closer to the mat. Do not tilt the top of your head into the mat, or press your neck and chin down.

14 Using imagery with exercise

Instead of making a shape or doing a movement by thinking about *how* you move, try visualising a sensation or an image. Imagining a feeling or picturing an activity can often help us access our deeper muscles and coordinate more easily. For example, when stretching your leg away from your hip, imagine someone is holding your foot and pulling it away from your body; or bring your arms together as if embracing a friend. We can breathe out, using our abdominals from the pubic bone up as if squeezing a tube of toothpaste from the bottom of the tube to the top, at the same time narrowing the waist as if zipping up a pair of tight trousers.

Visualising increasing *length* between specific body parts helps coordinate movements and achieve complex muscle work without over-focusing on specific muscles. Visualise your head lengthening away from your neck, or widening the back of your pelvis to release tension. Imagining lines of movement between related body parts contributes to connecting the muscles and improves coordination, while using imagery or visualisation can improve the precision and flow of the movement.

A gentle warm-up

The exercises presented in this section are very safe for most people. Follow the guidelines that precede each exercise carefully. It is a good idea to read the exercise descriptions out loud to yourself a few times before you attempt them. Practise the exercises with a progressive focus on the principles: first awareness, then alignment, breathing, the centre, *then* concentrate on getting the right muscles to work with precision. Do not just make shapes; move with coordination. Progress to the more complex work in Part III when you have developed a stronger connection between your mind and your body. Being persistent will help you improve both health and well-being—whatever shape you are in, whatever your age.

If you are very fit, try these gentle exercises after you have done a hard workout and are physically weary; in this state it is easier to find balanced motor control and connect to the right muscles, because the strong muscles are less likely to take charge.

Exercising in the supine position—supported rest position

Remember the more bits of your body are on the floor being supported, the less your body has to work to hold itself in relaxed natural alignment. Lying flat on your back with the legs stretched out straight may place strain on your lower back, as the pull of the leg and hip muscles makes it curve up away from the floor. Lying on your back with your knees bent and feet flat on the floor in the constructive rest position allows your back to relax toward the floor and encourages a natural spinal alignment, even though the lower body and legs are not fully at rest.

The supported rest position is also a very safe place to start to exercise, and is used frequently in modern Pilates. If you want to completely relax the body when lying on your back the legs may have to be supported. It is often recommended that the legs be supported bent at right angles, by resting the calves on a chair or similar, but in this position the knees tend to flop apart. To avoid this I developed the open supported rest position, using triangular pillows large enough to support the legs, allowing them to dangle with the feet off the ground, and thus letting the lower back relax. You can improvise with firm pillows, or by resting your lower legs over a low table with a pillow under your calves. The thighs should be held at an open angle, not directly above the hips.

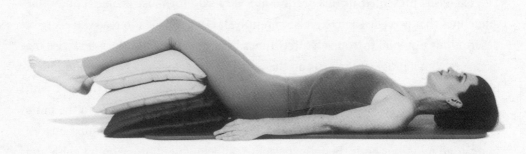

These first exercises can all be done with the legs in either the supported rest position or the constructive rest position.

15 Starting to move

You need a space large enough for an exercise mat, a few pillows and a long belt or scarf near at hand.

Lie in supported or constructive rest position and wobble your feet, gently rocking and wriggling your body into a comfortable position. Focus your awareness on yourself. Think and feel to find neutral spine and a relaxed body alignment. Say hello to your body with the breathing exercises. Then do these simple 'pre-Pilates' exercises, based on Eve Gentry's work.

HEAD ROLLS

Aim:

To create awareness of any neck and head tension, to relax and unwind neck and shoulders, and to increase awareness of the weight of the head.

To start, lie in constructive rest position, resting your head on a small pillow if your neck is tense.

Inhale and focus your awareness on how heavy your head feels, then begin to exhale and let your head roll gently to the side as you continue to exhale. After a slight pause inhale and gently return your head to the centre or upright position.

Repeat 4 times on each side, alternating from one side to the other.

Visualisation:

Your head is moving as though a weight is attached to your earlobe is drawing your head down, then the weight slips off and allows your head to return to centre.

Points of caution:

Take care not to turn your head too far or to force any twisting movement.

SHOULDER SHRUGS

Aim:

To relax and stretch between the spine and shoulder blades helping to reduce tension in the neck, stretching the rhomboids, and learning not to use the neck as you exercise.

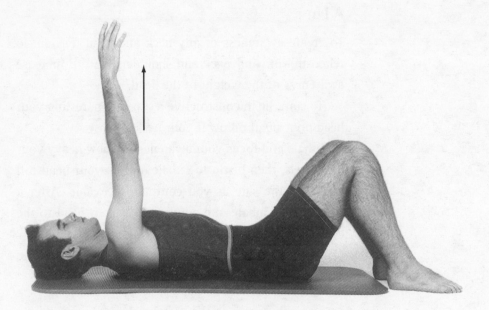

To start, lie in constructive rest position with a neutral spine. Raise one arm straight to the ceiling, perpendicular to the floor, palm inwards. Begin to inhale and stretch the raised arm toward the ceiling, letting your shoulder slide up and away from your spine, as you continue to inhale. Exhale and rest your shoulder back on the mat in a shrugging motion.

Repeat 4 times on each side, then repeat.

Visualisation:

Your heavy arm is reaching for the ceiling, as though a string tied to your wrist is being pulled up and relaxed.

Points of caution:

Take care to use only the pectoral muscles (upper chest to arm muscle) and front deltoid to lift the arm toward the ceiling, not the muscles of the neck and opposite shoulder, or your back.

Variation:

When you feel comfortable working with one arm raised, lift both arms to the ceiling and alternate the shrugging movements.

SINGLE LEG SLIDES

Aim:

To help gently connect and work your abdominal muscles, supporting and stabilising the centre, and separating the action of holding the abdominals from moving the leg.

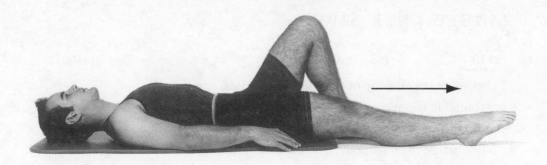

To start, lie in constructive rest position, focusing on your centre. Inhale, then begin to exhale and slide one leg along the mat, reaching your foot away from your pelvis. As you continue to exhale, narrow your waist and support your pelvis. Inhale, and slowly return your leg to the start position. Keep the upper body relaxed.

Repeat 5 times on one leg, then 5 times the other side.

Visualisation:

Your abdominals are drawing up from your pubic bone just as much as your leg is reaching away from your pelvis.

Points of caution:

Take care to start the movement with abdominal connection to the centre. Do not let your hips tilt or move with the movement of your leg. Keep a neutral spine with the back relaxed on the mat especially when the leg is straight.

Variation:

When you have a good connection with your abdominals, repeat the exercise alternating the sliding leg.

SINGLE KNEE SIDE

Aim:

To help with lateral sway or side control of pelvis, and to start building connections with the side of the waist (the oblique abdominals).

To start, lie in constructive rest position, focusing on

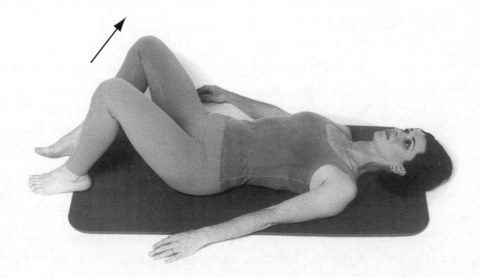

your centre. Inhale, as you exhale, gently move one knee out to the side and toward the floor, without moving your pelvis or feet. The intent is to move only the leg, holding your pelvis still with your abdominals. Return to start position, knees evenly to the ceiling, mentally checking you are still in neutral spine. Inhale to repeat.

Repeat 5 times on each side, then repeat.

Visualisation:

You have a very full bowl of soup on your stomach. You must not tip it or let it spill.

Points of caution:

Take care not to use your other leg as a counterbalance, (it is meant to stay still) or to grip the front of your hip to hold the pelvis still. Move the knee to the side only as far as you can while keeping your pelvis still. Don't be surprised if you can move your knee only a small distance at first. As you gain better control of your abdominals and stabilise your centre you will be able to move your knee further toward the floor.

16 The shoulder

Retaining a good postural alignment of our limbs while we are exercising is important. The upper body, shoulders, arms and head need to sustain a neutral alignment, while being careful not to overwork or help when we move the legs.

It is difficult at first to become aware of good arm and shoulder alignment, due partly to the complex nature of the shoulder joint and partly to the range of movement possible with your arms. The shoulder–arm joint is only a partial socket, with the rotator cuff muscles helping to hold the shoulder to the body (unlike the hip joint, which is a complete ball and socket joint).

The shoulder–arm complex attaches to the fixed skeleton (the spine) via the inner end of the clavicle, being otherwise 'free-floating' and connected to the skeleton by a complex array of muscles, some of which attach to the trunk. The components of the shoulder are the shoulder blade (scapula), the collarbone (clavicle) and the upper arm (humerus). All arm movements tend to involve the scapula and clavicle. If the scapula is over-involved in arm movements it causes all sorts of problems for that area.

Finding good shoulder alignment

Standing or sitting in front of a mirror, extend your right arm forward and then up toward the ceiling, then down. Is there space between your neck and the raised arm, or is your shoulder moving up toward your ear? Bring your arm down, then try raising your arm again, and imagine your shoulder blade sliding down and out toward the back of the armpit. This will create space between the arm and neck. Now try moving your arm just by moving the shoulder, as if they are all of a piece. Can you separate the different ways of moving the arm? If you can only move the shoulder and arm together then the joint is not working as it should. To reach your arm above your head your shoulder blade needs to slide out of the way of the top of your arm, although you can reach further upwards if the shoulder blade elevates at the end of the movement.

The arm and shoulder need to be able to work both separately and together, in smooth gentle rhythms, so as not to injure or strain the area. Many injuries to

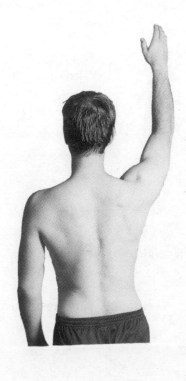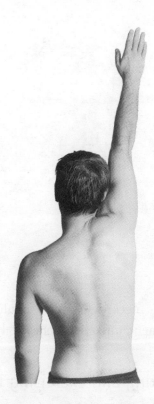

this area happen gradually and we may be unaware that we are incorrectly over-working muscles for many years.

The shoulder blade (scapula) floats freely on the back of the ribs, and the muscles of the shoulder joint are all attached to the scapula. We need to be able to hold and stabilise the scapula in order to freely move the arm and not overwork the deep supporting shoulder muscles, the rotator cuff muscles. Coordination of this complex joint is vital, but very difficult.

The scapula is muscularly suspended from the base of the skull and neck and connected to the lateral ribs and the mid- and lower thoracic spine. If one group of muscles underworks, another group of muscles will try and do their work as well. For example, if the lower outside muscles do not do their job (particularly the serratus anterior), the trapezius, rhomboids and other upper scapular muscles come into play. The body knows it has to hold the scapula, otherwise the arm cannot move properly. Additionally, if the upper scapular muscles get very strong, possibly by over-helping in breathing or constantly hunching the shoulders in a fixed posture, they will happily continue to overwork. Eventually we are left with

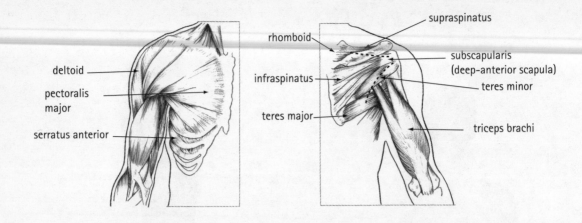

Anterior muscles of the shoulder   *Posterior muscles of the shoulder*

chronic neck and upper shoulder tightness and, eventually, pain, restricted movement, often headaches and other problems.

Relaxing and exercising the shoulders

To retrain the shoulders we need to find out what is overworking, then encourage it to let go—but overworked muscles will not let go unless other more appropriate muscles have started working. Generally the upper shoulder muscles overwork and the lower side shoulder muscles underwork. When we breathe we need to ensure that we primarily use our centre to breathe, rather than lifting the shoulders in siphon breathing.

ARM FLOATS

Aim:

To connect shoulder and arm movement (the humero-scapular rhythm). Relaxing the upper shoulder muscles and separating the arm movement with the shoulder supporting and lengthening.

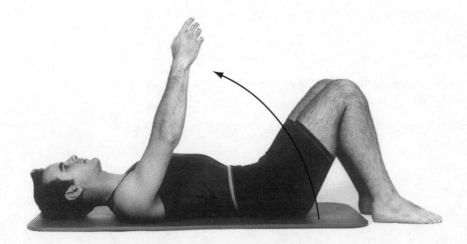

To start, lie in the constructive rest position with your arms resting by your sides and thumbs uppermost (to the ceiling). Inhale, relaxing neck and shoulders; as you exhale raise one arm up toward the ceiling very slightly drawing the shoulder blade down. Inhale again and pause, with arm to the ceiling. Exhale as you relax your arm back down onto the floor.

Repeat 5 times on one side, then repeat with the other arm.

Visualisation:

Your arm is the pencil attached to a geometry compass. You are tracing a quarter-circle with the pencil and holding the top of the compass with the muscles of the body.

Points of caution:

Take care not to elevate the shoulder with the arm, either by lifting it off the floor or up toward your neck, or to tense the opposite hip, or the chest.

ALTERNATING ARM OVERHEAD

Aim:

To help you lift your arm overhead without compressing or lifting the shoulder or using the neck muscles.

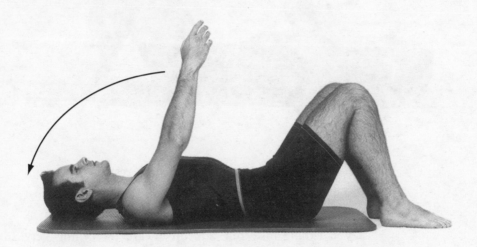

To start lie in constructive rest position, both arms raised toward the ceiling with both shoulder blades relaxed on the floor. As you exhale, reach one arm overhead and one down to the floor by the hip. Inhale and return to start position, with both arms up to the ceiling. Use your abdominal muscles to ensure the ribs on the same side do not lift with your arm. Aim to isolate the arms by stabilising your shoulder and drawing it towards the side of your waist. In this way the arms can move freely away from the stabilised centre.

Repeat 8 times, alternating the arms.

Visualisation:

You are holding a fragile flower between your lower ribs. As your arm goes overhead, carefully hold the flower firmly between your ribs.

Points of caution:

Take care to draw the shoulderblade down the back as your arm goes overhead. Do not let your ribs or spine lift.

ARM SLIDES

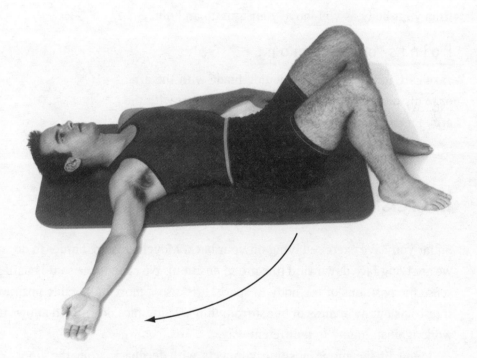

Aim:

To relax the shoulder joint and hold the scapula open while moving the arms apart sideways.

To start, lie in constructive rest position with your arms by the side of your body, thumbs uppermost. Inhale. As you exhale, slide one arm softly along the floor away from the hips with the palm to the ceiling, extended from the shoulder. Reach away from the body.

Only open the arm as far as you can while keeping the shoulderblade still. You may feel a stretch down through your arm. Inhale and relax the arm. Exhale, dragging the arm back to the start position next to the hips.

Repeat 8 times, then repeat with the other arm.

Visualisation:

Someone is pulling your shoulderblade out and away from your body as you move your arm up and out.

Points of caution:

Take care not to move the shoulderblade with the arm, or to distort the body while trying to reach out with the arm. Ensure that head and neck are relaxed.

17 Exercising in the prone position

So far you have exercised lying on your back. Movements are harder to do when we are lying face downward (the prone position). We cannot see so it is harder to sense the positions of the body in space. It is also a more vulnerable position as it restricts our awareness of our surroundings. Lying face downward allows us to work against gravity in a different way.

Lying in the prone position connects with feedback from the floor. With gravity acting against the abdominals more effort is required to work the centre. In this position you can feel whether your legs and buttocks are helping, or whether the upper body is elevating the chest unnecessarily. Placing pillows under your lower ribs and stomach may be more comfortable for your neck, shoulders and back.

Some of the exercises in this group were developed in England in the late 1970s and early 1980s specifically for dancers, and were done with weights, with the legs as turned out as possible. I have modified them to make them more appropriate for general use.

Points of caution:

Do not do these exercises if your back is very sore. Turning over from the prone position is extremely hard when you have severe low back problems. On pages 100–5 there are similar exercises done on all fours kneeling, that are kinder for the back.

STOMACH LIFTS

Aim:

To help connect with the centre, particularly the lower abdominals. Working against gravity improves awareness of upper body tension.

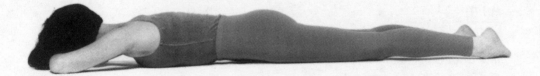

To start, lie on your stomach with elbows bent and hands resting on top of each other under your forehead. Your legs are resting, relaxed, with the heels to the outside (internally rotated) so there is no tension in your buttocks. Inhale, expanding right down to the pelvic floor and, broadening the abdominals to the floor, be aware of the back and rib cage expanding. Then exhale by lifting the abdomen upward from the pubic bone towards the waist. Drawing the lower abdomen up, without using other muscles, may seem hard at first as there is no joint action which assists with this movement. Inhale to repeat. Ensure that your head stays relaxed on your hands throughout the action.

Repeat 10 times.

Visualisation:

You are drawing in your lower abdominals as if you are zipping up a pair of tight trousers.

Points of caution:

Take care not to grip the buttocks together, lift the lower ribs off the floor, press your arms to the floor or raise your head.

DIAMOND PRESS

Aim:

To help you support your abdominals as you extend the mid thoracic area, protect the lumbar spine and connect your lower shoulder girdle.

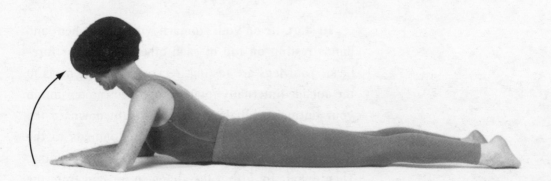

To start, lie prone. Make a diamond shape with your arms to frame your face on mat, with your fingertips just touching. Inhale. As you exhale press down on your forearms and hands, support and lift your lower stomach muscles, lift your upper body, shoulders, neck and head so as to stretch your mid-back above the waist, with your upper spine lengthened. Draw your shoulders down the sides of the body towards your waist.

Repeat 8 times.

Visualisation:

You are reaching the top of the head away from the base of your spine as though you are curving the upper body like the bow of a ship.

Points of caution:

Take care not to let go of the lower abdominals and thus overuse your lower back. Curve from the lower ribs, leaving the lower ribs softly on the floor. Ensure that your shoulders draw down and out and are not pinched together. Relax the buttocks and legs.

SINGLE LEG LIFT

Aim:

To use the hamstrings and extend the leg without bending the lower back, while supporting the centre.

To start, lie on your stomach, arms bent up so that

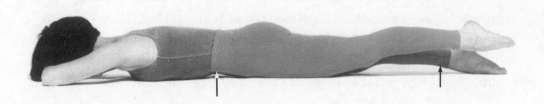

you can rest your forehead on your hands, with legs softly drawn together with heels touching. Inhale. As you exhale support your stomach with your abdominal muscles, then raise one leg slightly off the mat with softly pointed toes.

Repeat 5 times on each side.

Visualisation:

Someone is pulling your leg away from the pelvis.

Points of caution:

Take care not to sink the lower abdominals down as you lengthen the leg away. Do not turn out the legs. Check whether the shoulder opposite the raised leg is helping (it should not be) and keep the shoulders even.

18 The helpful body

Separating, moving and holding

The muscles both hold body parts still and move us around. If a group of muscles is asked to do both at once, confusion in the muscles is inevitable. We need to separate the holding work from the moving work. Our bodies try to be 'helpful' by letting the strong muscles always work.

If a muscle is given conflicting instructions, to hold still and move at the same time, it may seize up and compress the joint involved. Eve Gentry introduced the term 'joint release' into the Pilates vocabulary to indicate that joints were to float rather than being locked into position, as Pilates originally recommended. The sensation of floating, rather than locking, allows you to separate the moving part from the holding body area, and connects with the feeling of lengthening as you strengthen your body. If we reach away from the centre of the body, rather than pulling the body tight and hard, there will be no jarring or compression of the joint. We can use our muscles to create space in our joints rather than squashing them, thus helping to prevent joint injuries and perhaps reducing the incidence of degenerative changes in the joints. Our joints are very slow to repair as they have a very poor blood supply.

This group of exercises are done in the supine position.

SINGLE KNEE FLOATS

Aim:

To help keep the torso held in the centre without gripping the hip flexors or compressing the hip joints. This slightly increases the challenge to the abdominal muscles as they try to keep the centre firm.

To start, lie in the constructive rest position. Inhale and find neutral spine. Begin to exhale, floating the leg in its bent position toward the ceiling, keeping the hip securely on the floor and the lower back in supported neutral position. Inhale, with the knee pointing to the ceiling and your lower leg parallel to the ceiling, then exhale and float the leg back to the ground, separating the moving leg from the supported body.

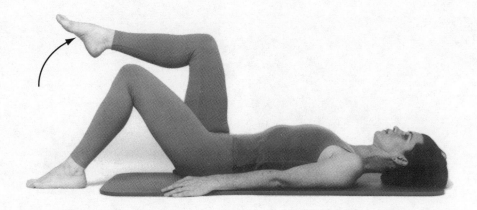

Visualisation:

The thigh is wafting up toward the chest as though you are gently waving a fan.

Variation:

You can change the rhythm and speed up the breathing, exhaling as you bring the leg up and inhaling as the leg goes down to the ground.

Points of caution:

Take care to keep the hip bones even and keep the front of the hip relaxed. Do not let the hip bone on the opposite side of the moving leg lift up.

SINGLE KNEE STIRS

Aim:

To help separate the torso and pelvis, holding firm in the centre, encouraging the leg to move fluidly in the hip socket with a released joint.

To start, lie in constructive rest position, then lift the right knee toward the ceiling, so that the thigh is vertical

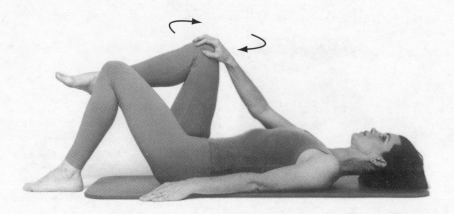

(points directly to the ceiling). Hold the right knee with the right hand and use the arm to assist in the circling of the knee to get the feeling of relaxation in the front of the hip joint. Draw a circle with the knee, keeping the pelvis still by using the abdominal muscles so that only the leg moves. Keep the circle very small to begin with.

Breathe out as you circle away from the body. Inhale as the leg comes towards the body.

Repeat 6 times both ways (with each leg).

Visualisation:

You are stirring a bowl of porridge or making gravy— your thigh is the spoon and your pelvis the bowl or pot.

Points of caution:

Keep the hip supported via the centre, with no circling movement in the torso. Relax the neck and shoulders. Do not grip with the front of the thigh.

SINGLE KNEE CIRCLES

Aim:

To further increase our ability to separate the torso and the centred pelvis from the moving leg.

To start, lie in constructive rest position and raise one leg toward the ceiling, knee bent at a right angle and toes softly pointed, while keeping the pelvis and spine aligned on the floor, arms resting by your side. Keep the leg with the foot resting on the floor aligned with your hip. Place your hands lightly in your hips.

Inhale: As you exhale, trace a circular shape with the raised leg going across the body first, then back down

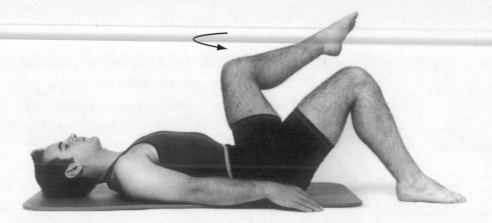

towards the floor and slightly outward, completing the circle by bring your leg up toward the ceiling. Inhale as your leg comes up. Continue the circle, exhaling as your leg moves around and away from the body.

Repeat the circle 4 times in the same direction, then circle 4 times the other way. Change legs, circling 4 times with the leg going across the body and 4 times in the outward direction. As you get stronger increase the repetitions to 6 times in both directions.

Visualisation:

Feel the relaxation in the moving leg, like a slowly rotating fan.

Points of caution:

Take care to relax the upper body and neck. Keep the hip bones even and still, with your centre engaged.

Variation:

You can do a similar thing with the shoulder and arm so that the shoulder is not compressed. Keep in mind the need for the shoulder to hold a very steady position in relation to the arm.

19 Depth and three-dimensional alignment

We often forget about the sides of our bodies. Even when we look sideways in the mirror we tend to look only at the outline we make with the front and back of the body. Our bodies have depth and space, with muscles wrapping around and through them. This allows us to move and reach out. If we had only front and back muscles, our ability to move and grasp things would be severely limited.

Alignment is not just linear and symmetrical—we have spiral muscle connections that let us move in a much more complex way. Spirals and twists are the most complex coordinated moves the body makes, the most important and the most vulnerable to strain and injury. How often as we turn over in bed do we feel a 'twinge'? Or getting out of the car or picking something off the floor? All these spiral movements are an ordinary part of life. In fact we rarely make a move that does not have a spiral component.

Diagonal connections

Most of us are either right or left handed. Being 'handed' in body terms means that we are better at finely coordinated movement with one hand and arm than with the other. We write and grasp better with that hand, for example. The opposite arm and shoulder are usually the strong 'holding' side, helping us to hold still and make the complex movements. The same goes for our legs. If you go to jump over something, or kick a ball, unconsciously you will use one leg to lead the action and the opposite hip and leg to help, hold and support. (This division of activity may be exaggerated in cases of scoliosis). Handedness and a degree of asymmetry are normal, but if we are too asymmetrical we will not be in balance. The torso responds to handedness so that one side of your abdominals is usually stronger than the other side; the same applies to the back.

Connecting internally with the sides of the body is usually a new experience but one vital for balance and alignment. When you lie on your side and relax, gravity rests your head on the floor and your waist droops to the floor, while the shoulders and pelvis support your spine in a lateral curve. Exercising in this position may be of great benefit for some back problems, assisting in creating lateral connections and encouraging the oblique and lateral abdominals to work.

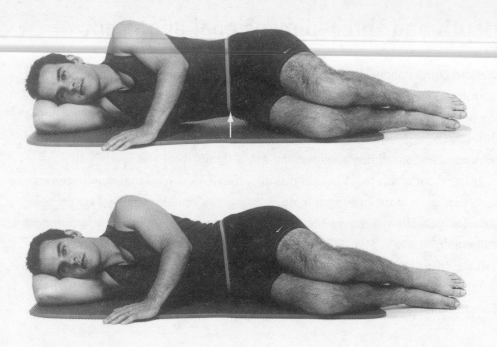

Lying on your side can be a very comfortable position. If you have back, shoulder or pelvic problems, however, it can be very awkward unless your pelvis and your spinal alignment are supported. This can be done by putting pillows between your knees, and under your waist and head if necessary.

SIDE LIE BREATHING

Aim:

To sustain neutral alignment in the spine and connect with the lateral abdominal muscles.

To start, lie on your side with the knees bent, feet in line with your pelvis, and your body lengthened out. You can put your lower arm or a pillow under your head for neck support. If you have a sore lower back or pain across the back of the pelvis, put a pillow between your knees. This helps with the lower body alignment

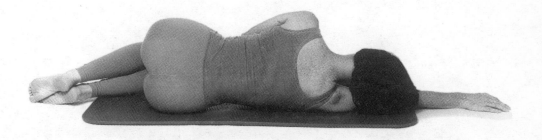

and can be an excellent 'rest' position for some low back problems.

Inhale, and expand the ribs and waist down into the floor. As you exhale, narrow the waist and try to lift the lower side of the waist off the floor and up towards the ceiling. You probably will not be able to lift the waist off completely at first. Inhale, relax and expand your waist and ribs sideways.

Repeat 6 to 8 times on each side.

Visualisation:

A string attached to the lower side of the waist is pulling it up, as though you are lifting your navel to the ceiling.

Points of caution:

Take care not to use your leg, clench your buttock muscles or elevate your shoulder muscles. Remember, you want to use only the stomach muscles to lift your waist.

LATERAL CLAMS

Aim:

This exercise is a progression from side lie breathing; it increases the work of the side abdominals and works the top outer side of the thigh.

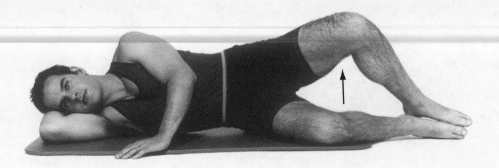

To start, lie on your side with knees bent at 45° to your body, feet together in a line with the body.

Inhale, expanding the lower ribs and abdomen and feeling the side of the waist on the floor. Exhale, lifting the abdomen off the floor, using your centre. Then raise your top knee toward the ceiling without lifting the foot from its resting place on top of the other foot. Keep your body supported and centred, with the pelvis perpendicular to the floor. Inhale and relax your knee down, resting it back on the lower leg.

Repeat 6 to 8 times on each side.

Visualisation:

Your leg is like a door opening and shutting against a fixed doorframe. Or, from the name of the exercise, your legs are the shell of a clam or an oyster opening and shutting.

Points of caution:

Take care not to use your shoulders or move your waist. Also ensure that you do not roll your pelvis back as you move your leg. Focus on the muscles that outwardly rotate the leg, the buttock muscles.

SIDE SINGLE LEG LIFT

Aim:

To use the side and hip muscles more strongly, with the leg out straight in a line with the body and the focus more on the side hip muscles. As the lever (outstretched leg) is longer, it takes more work to keep the pelvis secure at right angles to the floor.

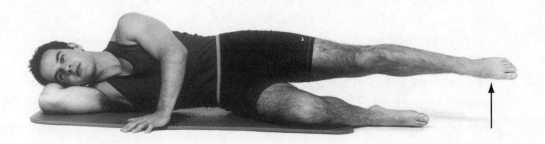

To start, lie in side lie position with the lower leg resting bent on the floor. The top leg is straight with the foot on the floor in line with the body. Inhale. As you exhale, reach with the top leg and lift it so that it is parallel to the floor, with a softly pointed foot.

Repeat 6 to 8 times each side.

Visualisation:

You are reaching away with the lifted leg to touch the far wall, rather than up to the ceiling.

Points of caution:

Take care not to sink the waist to the floor and tilt the pelvis. The aim is to move the leg without changing the alignment of the body.

Variation:

Lift your leg and move it in 4 very small circles before returning it to the floor. Exhale as you circle.

20 Connecting and disconnecting muscles

So far we have been isolating the upper and lower body work so as to be very specific in employing movements that connect with the less-used (or mis-used) muscles.

After practising the side lie work you should have some sense of which is your strong holding side, and which is the less connected side. But sometimes the body complicates the spirals of work so that it has the upper body holding on one side and the lower body holding *on the same side*, so that we become very one-sided physically. (Might this reflect an emotional state as well?) To make cross-spiral connections without unnecessary tension, we need to connect the right upper body with the left lower body and vice versa.

DIAGONAL KNEE PRESS

Aim:

To help connect the diagonals of the body; to become more aware of which spiral holding pattern is the strongest and therefore the most frequently used. It also helps create an awareness of which extra muscles are overworking in twisting and spiral movements.

To start, lie on your back with legs bent in supported rest position. Cross one ankle over the opposite knee, and relax the knee of the crossed leg towards your navel. Place your opposite hand on the inside of the lifted knee.

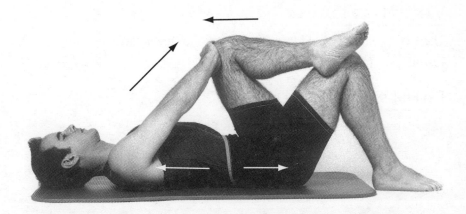

Inhale and check your alignment. As you exhale, press your knee into your hand and resist the pressure back through the hand and arm. Make sure the pressure of your knee back into the hand is equal to the pressure down the arm. Be aware of a circle of work down through your arm, through your shoulder and across your chest, diagonally to your abdomen and opposite hip, and up the inside thigh of the lifted leg to the knee. Sense an even amount of work connecting your arm to opposite leg without shortening the distance between the shoulder and the hip.

Try to feel your back lengthen along the floor as though the work at the front of the body is enabling the inside of the spine to stretch out. Make a careful mental check that the opposite working diagonal is not helping. Relax the arm resting on the floor and soften the leg that is supporting the lifted leg, particularly at the front of the hip. Exhale and relax the effort of work, while gently keeping the connection between your hand and knee.

Repeat 4 times on one side then 4 times on the other. Repeat the sequence again.

Visualisation:

The two points of shoulder and hip are moving apart, just like stretching toffee.

Points of caution:

Take care not to use your neck and head.

SUPINE BACK RELAX

Aim:

To relax your back and legs.

To start, lie in the constructive rest position. Bend both knees up to your chest, one at a time, keeping the knees slightly apart. Place both hands on your knees, inhale, then pull gently in toward your chest. As you exhale, think of lengthening your spine along the floor. Inhale, and relax the knee slightly away from the chest.

Repeat the gentle stretch a few times.

Kneeling

Being up on all fours, like a baby learning to crawl, assists in establishing co-ordination. Being on all fours is a great way to make connections between the upper and lower body, and helps to re-establish the cross-spirals of the body. It is a safe alternative position for some of the prone work, but can be hard on the knees and wrists.

In this position we can practice abdominal exercises such as stomach lifts. It is more work for the abdominals and you need to make sure you hold your shoulders in supported alignment.

FOUR-POINT KNEELING TO CAT STRETCH

Aim:

To connect upper and lower abdominal supporting muscles.

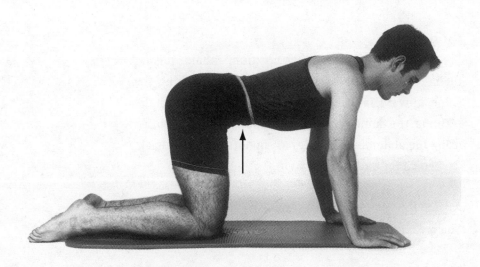

Four-point kneeling

To start, take up a square kneeling position on all fours with knees slightly apart, thighs vertical and your hands are placed, usually slightly wider than shoulder-width apart, so that your shoulders are in alignment. Your feet should be relaxed. The spine should be approximately parallel to the floor. Inhale and expand the waist. Exhale and narrow the waist, lifting the stomach to the spine without moving your spine or your hips, keeping the spine in neutral alignment.

Repeat 10 times.

Visualisation:

You are blowing up balloons as you exhale.

Points of caution:

Take care not to arch your lower back down toward the floor or lift the spine to the ceiling when the stomach lifts.

Variation:

Rest on your forearms if you have sore wrists.

Cat stretch
Stay in the 4-point kneeling position. Inhale, raising the mid back to the ceiling, flexing and stretching the spine upward, and breathing into the back. Exhale, relaxing the spine down in a supported neutral spine, using the abdominal muscles to support the lower back.

Repeat 8 times.

Visualisation:

You are a cat lifting and stretching her spine after a rest.

REST POSITION

This position is similar to yoga's 'pose of the child'. You should only attempt it if your knees are pain free.

Aim:

To relax the spine and take tension out of neck and shoulders.

To start, kneel on all fours and inhale. As you exhale, sink your body back and down to rest between your thighs. Softly reach out your arms on the floor in a V shape and rest your forehead on the floor.

Remain in the position for 6 to 10 slow breaths.

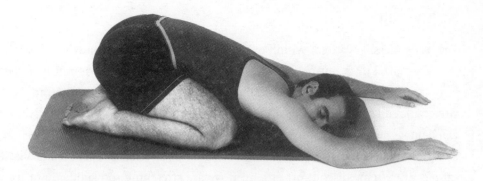

Visualisation:

The weight of your body is sinking into the floor; the tension is running out of your back down into the floor.

Points of caution:

Take care if you have sore knees or pain in the lower back; you can modify the rest position by placing a large pillow between your body and thighs.

21 Relaxing through stretching

It is important that you stretch safely. Be aware of which muscles you are stretching, and be careful not to accidentally stretch an adjacent body area. Unfortunately, just as strong muscles always work too much, so also do flexible body parts always tend to overstretch. It is also quite easy to get in a muddle about what is tense and what is tight. If you try to stretch muscles that are tense, you tend to 'tie them in knots' so that they become tight. Forcing a stretch in tight muscles can injure the muscle. Tense muscles are often tight, so that relaxing, breathing and deliberately letting go of tightness is the first thing to do.

Many of the previous exercises can be used to help relax a tense or tight muscle. The supported rest position, with lots of pillows underneath the legs, is a good place to begin the process of letting go.

Stretching

There is a message system within our bodies that lets us know how much strain or stress is placed on a muscle and thus assists with injury protection. It is based on sensors in muscles, joints and tendons called proprioceptors. It is good to feel the stretch in a muscle, but not good to overstretch it or stretch it too suddenly, as this can damage both muscle and tendons. The two stretch reflexes that we need to be aware of and listen to, the golgi tendon reflex and the stretch reflex, tell us via sensations of extreme discomfort or pain if we are stretching too suddenly or for too long (see page 48 on reflexes).

It is important to remember that the body is more elastic if it is warmed up a bit by doing gentle stretches. Leaping out of bed in the morning and immediately getting stuck into very vigorous stretches may be harmful.

KNEELING HAMSTRING STRETCH

Aim:

To help stretch out the front of the thigh (the quadriceps) and the top of the back of the thigh (the hamstring).

To start, kneel on all fours. Bring your right leg forward between your hands so that you are resting on the right foot at the front and the left knee and shin at

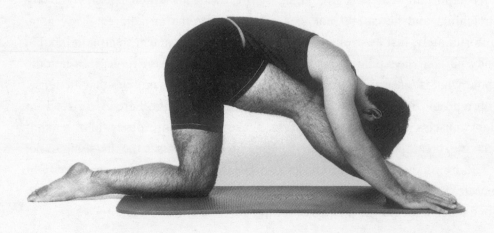

the back. The front foot should be slightly forward of the knee so that the distance between it and the knee on the floor is greater than the length of your raised thigh.

To begin the stretch, rest your body on the raised right thigh and lean gently forward with the body over the right knee, lengthening the hips away from the front of the left thigh and stretching the left quadriceps. Rest there for four breaths. Then tilt your body down and back towards the floor, slightly straightening the front leg. Try to draw the top of your head towards your front heel. Make sure that you keep your body touching your thigh the whole time, with the front knee next to your armpit, so that you lengthen both your spine and the right side of your body, stretching the right hamstring gently. Rest and sustain this hamstring stretch position for four breaths.

Repeat 4 times, going forward for the quadriceps stretch and back to stretch the hamstring, finishing in the 4-point kneeling position. Then change legs and repeat with the left foot forward.

Points of caution:

Take care not to curve the spine up toward the ceiling in full stretch postion, or to let the thigh and body move apart. Avoid twisting the hips. Do not bounce the body or pull the leg to increase the stretch.

Repeat the rest position.

ARM OPENINGS

Aim:

To stretch the upper body making a gentle spiral, opening the chest, relaxing and stretching muscles from the chest to the arm.

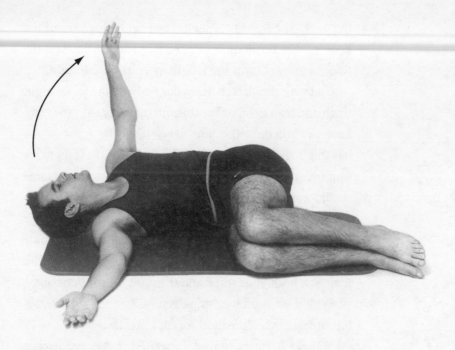

To start, lie on your side with your legs bent and together, knees at waist level. Extend your arms straight out in front of your body at shoulder level, resting them on the floor in a relaxed way, palms together.

Inhale. Open the top arm in an arc towards the ceiling, exhaling as you continue to open the arm out and down toward the floor behind you, still at shoulder level. Let your head move slowly with your arm. Your arm does not have to touch the floor; just relax it in the open position. Try to keep the neck long with a feeling of stretch across the upper chest.

Inhale, and return your arm in an arc to the front of your body, your head following the movement. Rest the moving hand back on the hand that has remained on the floor.

Repeat 5 to 10 times on each side.

Visualisation:

Your moving arm is like a frond on a palm tree, gently waving in the breeze.

Points of caution:

Take care to keep the knees well bent at hip level, with the lower body centred, and hips and legs still. Keep the moving arm relaxed, with soft fingers and wrist.

YAWN AND RELAX

Aim:

To finish off the basic mat programme.

To start, lie in the side lie position with the knees slightly bent. Inhale through the mouth, not the nose, deeply stretching out your jaw and opening your mouth as wide as possible to promote a yawn reflex. Stretch out the whole body, reaching your arms overhead and legs out, as you yawn. Inhale through your nose and exhale with a relaxed breath, like a sigh. Curl up into a soft foetal position, inhale gently through your nose and roll to the other side of your body. Exhale. Then inhale strongly through the mouth again, stretching and yawning, and repeat the sequence.

Repeat 2 or 3 times on each side.

Points of caution:

Take care to move slowly through the stretches. Rest a moment, lying on your side, before you get up. Only do the large inhale with the mouth open as you yawn, so as not to overbreathe.

22 Summary of basic mat programme

Each time you practise these exercises focus on a different aspect of the work.

- Remember a few principles at a time; move with focused awareness and neutral alignment.

- Try doing the exercises while focusing only on breathing and the centre.

- Move on to sensing more complex things, using your improved understanding of muscles.

- Coordinate your breathing with each movement.

- Lengthen out your body as the gradual process of mental and physical integration occurs.

- Relax chronically overworked muscles.

- Feel whether you are overusing your neck and face muscles, for example, perhaps your buttock and leg muscles, and work with precision.

- With persistence, good alignment and muscle recruit-ment will start to become habits in the body. These foundation exercises can be continued as long as you want. They will remain fresh as long as you vary the intention and the focus from time to time (even day to day). Use them to become aware of your body, and be patient with yourself as you improve your fitness and move toward sustainable good health.

The basic programme checklist

Supine

Breathing
Head rolls
Shoulder shrugs
Single leg slide
Single knee side

Arm floats to arms over head
Arm slides

Prone

Stomach lifts
Diamond press
Single leg lift

Supine

Single knee floats
Single knee stirs to single knee circles
Knee press
Back relax

Lateral

Side breathing
Clams
Side leg lift

Four-point kneeling

Breathing on all fours
Cat stretch
Rest position
Kneeling hamstring stretch

To finish—lateral

Arm openings
Yawn and relax

Part III

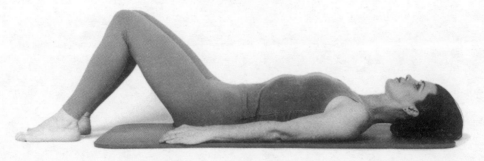

Safe fitness

In this section you build on your increasing knowledge of your body to improve strength, flexibility and quality of muscle control with additional information about the body and an intermediate level exercise programme. You need to have practised the basic programme at least three times a week for about six weeks before adding these exercises. As long as you have no injuries or painful areas, and are comfortable with the basic exercises, it is safe for you to continue straight on.

Read through the instructions a few times before you attempt the exercises. If you have any kind of chronic back and neck problems, you should not attempt exercises such as the curl up without the assistance of a qualified Pilates instructor. Gradually add one or two new exercises to your basic programme each week. Any pain or discomfort experienced during a new exercise, or even a couple of days after introducing the exercise, or a modification or variation, means that you should return to practising the more basic version of that exercise for a few weeks—but continue with the rest of the sequence. Re-introduce the more difficult variations when you feel stronger.

23 Muscles working together

New ideas

This section introduces further concepts relating to the body and re-introduces some of the original mat exercises in a modified form. The basic programme should be maintained, as part of warming up. You can include the exercises in this chapter after the kneeling hamstring stretch. Do arm openings then yawn and relax to finish. When you begin adding new exercises, you do not need to add them all at once. I suggest various sequences for a full programme on pages 183–6. You will find that many exercises have a progression, from an initial version to a more advanced version. After you have felt comfortable with the initial version for a couple of weeks begin to try some of the modifications. Go at your own pace, but remember—it is persisting with regular practice that gives lasting effects.

Some of these next ideas may seem rather complex. Do not be concerned. Anything really useful takes a while to integrate, but while this is happening your postural alignment will continue to improve and your fitness increase.

Having a good understanding of the complex workings of the body so that you can sense more accurately what is happening when you attempt more challenging work is important. The good thing is that once you reach that level of understanding you can mostly let your body be on autopilot (back to the analogy of driving a car).

Muscles working together

The body is made up of bones, ligaments, tendons, fascia and muscles, the internal organs (viscera), a neurological system that senses and advises the body what to do, and other support systems.

The bones are the internal support structure from which all of our soft tissue is suspended, attached and/or contained. We have many differently shaped bones, ranging from long and slender, like leg bones, to the small and variably shaped bones of wrist and ankle to the broad curved structure that is the pelvis.

Our bones move via joints of different types, such as the hinge joints of knee and elbow, or the ball-and-socket joints of hip and shoulder. The surfaces of the bones at a joint are coated with articular cartilage which allows the joint to variously glide, pivot or rotate, and helps absorb impact.

Ligaments both hold the joints together (sustain the joint structure) and allow them to move. They are relatively inelastic and if repeatedly overstretched become lax and unable to do their job properly. This can mean the joint becomes unstable. (They are often confused with tendons.) Muscles, tendons and ligaments hold the skeleton together, move the body and support soft tissues. We are interested in the skeletal muscles which (via tendons) attach to and move our bones and are the connections for the internal scaffolding of the body. The muscles can work (contract) in different ways to allow us to move. They can shorten and work (a concentric action), lengthen and work (eccentric action) or hold still (isometric contraction). They can also let go (relax) or be inhibited. The muscles are wrapped around with fascia, a 'wrap' which separates and surrounds and provides gliding connections for all soft tissue. The fascia forms thin slender bands or pathways across different muscles, creating slithery flowing spirals up and down, around and through the body (see Meyers 1999).

Types of muscle

Skeletal muscle can be divided into two basic types in terms of function, postural (or holding) and phasic-locomotor (or moving) muscle. They can also be divided into different types according to how they work, fast twitch and slow twitch muscle (there are also intermediate types). Fast twitch muscles tend to be large and short-acting, providing instant power or force, such as the quadriceps in the thigh and the biceps in the arm. Slow twitch muscles have the ability to work constantly at a low level and tend to be the deeper, more slender postural muscles such as transversus abdominis and the deep spinal muscles.

In modern Pilates work we tend to focus initially on the slow twitch postural muscles, as it is primarily these muscles that develop ingrained habits through either overtightness or atrophy.

How muscles work

Muscles work in groups and pairs, never in isolation. For example, when you bend your arm at the elbow, the muscle at the front of the upper arm (biceps brachii) shortens to pull the forearm towards the upper arm and your hand moves towards your shoulder. At the same time the muscle at the back of the upper arm (triceps) has to lengthen smoothly to allow the arm to bend. When one muscle of a pair is shortening and working (concentric action), the paired opposite muscle needs to be able to lengthen with a controlled release. If you reach your arm away from the shoulder with some resistance or weight, your muscles control the straightening by lengthening and working (eccentric action). The Pilates method places emphasis on this kind of action. If one muscle is shortened very quickly and powerfully, its paired opposite muscle lets go and relaxes with the reflex called reciprocal inhibition, which works to prevent injury.

Most exercise programmes focus on the muscles that create gross movement— but of equal importance are the muscles that hold still and allow you to move precisely, such as the muscles that allow you to bend your elbow without moving your whole body. These muscles act as postural holding muscles. When you bend your arm at the elbow, a group of muscles holds the top of the arm steady, letting you bring your arm (hand) to your shoulder rather than your shoulder to your arm. These muscles are acting as 'stabilisers'.

Thus, for every movement there is one group of muscles actively making the movement, another letting you do it, and another group holding the rest of the body still so that you can do the action without moving the rest of your body inappropriately. There are also additional muscles helping with the main action (synergists) and another diagonally opposed (or spiral) muscle (or group of muscles or parts of muscles) supporting and aligning the main muscles and allowing space to manoeuvre the joint. The joint aligning muscles commonly work in a spiral pattern contributing to stabilisation and the initiation of the opposing muscles' eccentric effort, and can be confused with the synergists.

The joint aligning muscles help protect the joint capsule by facilitating translation moves that allow space for glide and manoeuvring, so that on flexing and/or extending a joint there is minimal compression and an easy flow of movement.

Before a complex movement sequence takes place the parts of the body needed for the eccentric and stabilising work momentarily pause, with a slight softening of muscle tone or relaxation. Relaxation in this context does not mean everything turning to jelly—it is rather a slight letting go, a reduction of residual muscle tension, a sort of momentary aware restfulness. Mime artists exaggerate this 'prepare to move and pause' to portray a movement or effort in space when there is minimal spatial movement or real effort.

Sequence of movement

Prepare to move
- slight pause with relaxation (eccentric muscle preparation)

- recognition of correct initial stabilisers

- spiral joint aligning muscles engaged

Initiate movement
- slight eccentric then concentric work

- increase stabilisation

- continue movement under load (balance of concentric and eccentric work)

- stabilisers focus on eccentric as wel as concentric muscle attachments for smooth control, not just the concentric muscles (this is what allows for joint release in the following phase)

Peak of effort
- concentric muscles working strongly, stabilisers hold

- spiral joint spacing muscles work with eccentric and stabilising muscles

Prepare to move (to 'undo' movement) relax/pause
- concentric work becomes eccentric work

- stabilisers reduce effort

- coordination with unwinding joint spacing muscles

- relaxation with preparatory pause for next movement cycle

If we miss the prepare to move–relaxation–pause phase of a movement we recruit too many shortening muscles and compress the joint. When you have become familiar with the exercises and are practising a complete sequence, it is a good idea to plan a pause or space, with a full breath cycle, between each exercise. Always do this when you are in the start position for each new exercise, so that preparing to move is an integral part of the work.

In the previous section we focused on relaxing overused muscles, connecting with the central stabilisers, and maintaining bodily alignment. This focus becomes even more important when you are making your body work harder in the next sequence of exercises. You will be reducing the area that is stabilised, and increasing the effort (or work) by moving your limbs in broader ranges of movement, while supporting more of their weight. Accuracy and alignment are much harder to achieve when you are working progressively harder and faster. The body usually wants to recruit more large muscles rather than be muscle-specific. Working with aligned coordination and precision by initiating muscle-specific repose or relaxation is even more important with this more complex body work.

Muscle attachments and pathways

Muscles are made up of bundles of fibres like long tubes gathered together. A muscle fibre shortens equally over its whole length, but its action is also directly influenced by the stabilisers that act on the muscle. If one end is held firm the other end will move towards the fixed end. Since not all muscle fibres attach at exactly the same spot, some parts of a muscle tend to work more than others in particular actions, creating open or closed diagonals or spirals of work. This is particularly true of fan-shaped and multiple-attached muscles.

When a muscle travels over more than one joint (a two-joint muscle, such as the biceps brachii, rectus femoris or hamstrings), the action at either end or attachment is strongly influenced by how each end is held (by its stabilisers). Who is doing what to whom is very difficult to determine. Often we need to look elsewhere, perhaps at a distance from the action, to get some idea of what is happening to the body, particularly looking to the body's deeper muscles, and our main supporting area, the centre. Even though a muscle shortens over its whole length, when it works the way the muscle of action is held will affect whether it shortens toward one end or the other. Also, some muscles seem to selectively 'fire' small groups of bundles of fibres so that their angle of pull varies and only parts of the muscle appear to work.

A muscle may contribute to many different actions. Sometimes some parts of a single muscle appear to work in opposition to other parts of the same muscle, or to stabilise a movement. The key seems to be how a muscle is stabilised or held, and where the action of gravity and centre of balance are in relation to where the exertion of force is focused. Thus you may strain your elbow from overwork because of incorrect work in the shoulder, neck and torso, not just because the muscles of your elbow are weak. Or you may hurt your back because your abdominals are weak and your hip flexors or hamstrings are tight and short.

Muscles, or parts of them, fire in a sequence of work which lets us make complex movements, such as walking or sitting or typing on a keyboard, successfully. A sequence can have many successful variations. However, if the sequences a body has developed are stressed and overused, they begin to cause problems. This is particularly true if the lengthening muscle does not relax and pause at the beginning of the movement or if the stabilisers do not help correctly. An example is holding your back too rigidly, perhaps when sitting in an uncomfortable chair or using a computer mouse for long periods of time. It is rather like engaging the clutch incompletely when you drive a car. If you ride the clutch all the time it wears out.

We also want to have a range of strength: not just to be strong in one position, but to have strength right to the end of our range of movement with shifting stabilisation. This is known as 'dynamic support'. Many exercise programmes strengthen only within a short range, missing out on strengthening the muscles in their fully lengthened state or in eccentric muscle action. Muscles tend to tighten when we work them. Unless we try to keep them lengthened, and put effort into the eccentric phase of movement, they stay short.

24 Using our muscles

To exercise without causing injury we need to develop fine muscle control and muscle specificity, and balance the concentric or shortening work with eccentric or lengthening work, that is, only putting effort exactly where it is needed. The Pilates method's ability to achieve bodily economy and grace in movement comes from utilising the principles of always starting from the centre of the body and proceeding with a focus on minimal movement, with fine precision, for maximum effect, holding and supporting the correct parts of the body so that we only move or work specific muscles.

The often-attempted abdominal 'crunch' or 'curl' is a ready example of muscle use gone wrong. It is very easy to misuse or overuse many different muscles to make the curl shape. To bend or flex the body towards the legs when lying down, the muscles at the front of the body must shorten. They have to work concentrically to raise the weight of the body against gravity. The body knows that it is easiest to draw in close to the centre of the body, because the further the weight is away from the centre the more work is needed to make the shape. Thus we tend to compress the body on effort (the lazy way) if we use only the main (prime) moving muscle without the other helping and holding muscles.

Abdominal curl

When we do an abdominal crunch or curl in the old-fashioned way, we tend to scrunch up and squash the front of the body, neck and shoulders, using the upper legs. This compresses the joints of the spine, the ribs and the front of the hip, and the stomach pops up. If we do not lengthen as we strengthen, and work precisely from our whole centre, we will use only the vertical stomach muscle, the rectus abdominis, to achieve the curl. Then we have to use our hip flexors and buttock muscles to help hold the end of the rectus abdominis still and lift the legs. We end up crunching the lower back and putting a lot of pressure on the lumbar spine— which is not good for the back and can cause disc damage. It also overuses the hip flexors, particularly the psoas. The other three abdominals are underused.

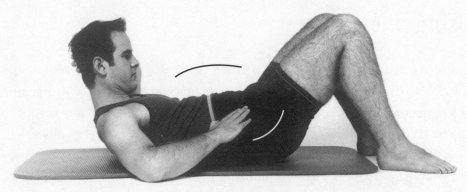

Incorrect curl up

The hip flexors are made up of three muscles or muscle groups, the combined iliacus and psoas major and minor, the quadricep muscle (rectus femoris), and the sartorius, which all attach to the leg and the pelvis. The iliopsoas then proceeds through the body on the internal bowl of the pelvis and up to the spine, attaching at the lumbar vertebrae. The hip flexors are easily overused, along with the rectus abdominis and the upper gluteus maximus. If these muscles are overworking it means the centre is not working properly.

This exercise is not suitable for everyone, it is intended for those who are moderately fit, with no back or neck problems. The abdominal curl following the principles of the Pilates method will challenge your ability to use your centre appropriately, as well as clarify for you the need to reduce the leg and hip flexor work and other inappropriate muscle recruitment.

CURL UP

This exercise is the foundation for many traditional Pilates exercises, including the hundred, the double leg stretch, the teaser and the neck pull. Variations of it are often seen in gyms. Do not attempt the curl up if you have a sore neck or an upper or lower back problem.

The curl up is very difficult to do correctly because it is extremely easy to bring the wrong muscles into play. The hip flexors want to bring the body to the legs, and the leg muscles may want to grip the floor and do most of the work, rather than the abdominal muscles doing the work. The neck and upper chest muscles are also prone to overworking.

Aim:

To strengthen the centre, ensuring that the deep abdominals support and work correctly.

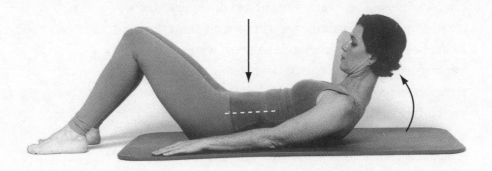

In fact, there are more don'ts for this exercise than dos.

To start, lie in constructive rest position, placing one hand on the back of your head with the other resting on your stomach.

Inhale gently and expand your waist. As you exhale, narrow your waist, articulate through your upper spine bending at the lower ribs. Leave your lower spine relaxed in neutral. Lift your head and shoulders far enough off the mat, initiating the movement with *all the abdominals*, so that you can comfortably look at your knees. Relax your body and head down as you inhale, uncurling from the centre.

Repeat 4 times with the same hand behind your head, then change arms and repeat 4 times.

Visualisation:

Your spine is lengthening as it curls up and the top of your head is reaching towards the ceiling. Imagine you are anchored into the middle of the pelvis, below the waist, like the base of a crane. Imagine you are squeezing a toothpaste tube with the muscles of the centre.

Points of caution:

Take care not to bring the pubic bone towards the ribs, and don't use your hip flexors or buttock muscles. Be careful not to pull the chin forward and down onto the chest. You want a lengthened curve with the effort focused on abdominal strength, with the wrap-around transversus and oblique muscles controlling the straight rectus abdominis so that the abdomen does not bulge as you curl up.

Extra care needs to be taken so the buttocks do not clench together, and the thighs must not grip. The lower and mid back should not press too firmly into the floor—neither tilting the pelvis back nor lifting the tailbone.

Variations:

Instead of resting your hand on your stomach, reach it toward the opposite knee and do a diagonal curl, with your head aligned with the reaching hand. Look towards the knee. This is considerably harder, and extra care is needed to ensure the opposite hip does not help.

As you get more confident with the correct muscle recruitment, you can modify your leg positions and lift and hold each leg up in the air, bent at right angles, as you reach towards it.

Traditional Pilates exercises based on the curl up are discussed in Chapter 38 (pages 198–201).

Applied posture and external forces: gravity

- Gravity acts on us at all times, though we are rarely aware of it.

- Whenever any part of the body is lifted off the floor the force of gravity tries to pull it back down.

- The further the lifted body part is taken from the centre, the harder the work to keep it off the ground.

- Gravity is responsible for activating our postural muscles.

- Posture is not static—we are always moving.

- Because the force of gravity follows a direct line or pathway through the body, in some exercises we need to be more than muscle-specific, to counter its effects—we need to be fibre-specific.

- Remember—turning down or reducing muscle work can be just as important as turning it on or increasing it.

25 Ways of centring with lengthened joints

The centre is that area of the body from the pelvic floor up to the lower ribs and thoracic diaphragm, with the abdominals supporting the lower spine and pelvic bowl. In working with the centre, we need to take into account the effect of gravity and the work of the lower pelvic stabilisers, the muscles of the legs that attach to the pelvis. These include the quadriceps, hamstrings, inside thigh muscles (adductors), buttock muscles and, most importantly, the hip flexors—the deep iliopsoas and rectus abdominis. These lower pelvic stabilisers are also our prime moving muscles, so they are used to doing a lot of work. When we exercise lying down these muscles can more readily relax.

The centre does not work in isolation. We have a 'ball' of muscles that surround and make up the perimeter of our centre, like an elasticised sausage. Below that central ball is a support structure that both interacts and is interwoven with it, our leg and buttock muscles. Unfortunately it is only too easy to overuse the leg and buttock muscles to help hold the pelvis and lower back upright, as well as the rest of the body. This is particularly true of much fast gym work and the most advanced traditional Pilates work. Overtraining and overdeveloping these big muscles can cause many problems, not just in the hips but also in the lower back. In particular, if we misuse the iliopsoas it can pull the lower back into an arch, compressing the discs and contributing to anterior hip problems. (The iliopsoas is the only muscle that travels from the upper centre through the lower centre and down to the thighs.)

Thus, when you work your stomach muscles strenuously and move your legs at the same time, make sure you are not overusing your buttock and thigh muscles. Think of the legs as a weight on the end of the abdominal muscles that the abdominals have to work against and help support, rather than allowing the leg and buttock muscles to do all the work supporting the pelvis. If you can make this change, then the Pilates centre really does become the centre of support.

Using this understanding you can perform increasingly difficult exercises without pain or discomfort or overworking inappropriate muscles.

Safe but strong

In the exercises so far we have primarily supported the body, legs and head on the mat, or kept the moving parts near to the centre of the body. To increase effort and muscle work for the centre we will now lift the legs off the floor so that their weight adds leverage or load to the body, particularly to the stomach. The important thing is to remember to still apply all the principles of the method—awareness or thinking of the muscles, focusing on the centre, lengthening and feeling the body connections. Forget about making shapes in the air.

Leg alignment

Our posture is affected by our leg alignment. Kendall identified the three basic leg alignments—knock-knees, bow legs and neutral—which describe the general bony alignment between the feet and the hips looked at from the front with the feet parallel. Your knees may come together or curve away from each other or make a straight line. The most functional is the straight (ideal) alignment, with knock-knees the most vulnerable to injury. When we straighten our legs it is important not to lock the knees back (hyperextend) but to draw the kneecaps up into

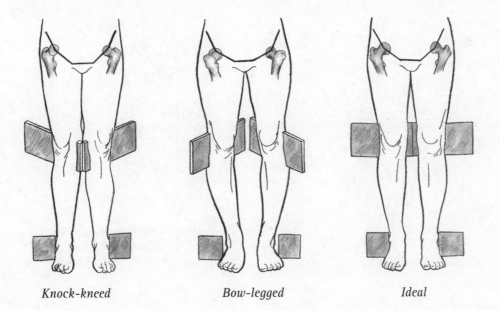

Knock-kneed   *Bow-legged*   *Ideal*

straight alignment. In this way, even if your bony alignment is not ideal your muscles are supporting a more functional position.

There are also different directional leg alignments, in which we turn our legs away from each other or towards each other. We can rotate our whole leg inward (internal rotation) and outwards (external rotation); a slightly turned-out leg stance is stronger than the legs parallel position. The martial arts use a slightly turned-out stance; extremely turned-out legs are synonymous with classical ballet.

Traditional Pilates worked primarily with moderately turned-out legs. The turned-out leg is easier to hold as we have extra holding and turning-out muscle power in the gluteus maximus and the external rotators, assisted by parts of the biceps femoris and iliacus muscles. In modern Pilates it is important to avoid both turning out and turning in of the legs, until you are comfortable with parallel leg alignment, to avoid recruiting inappropriate or unnecessary muscles. If the buttock muscles are very weak, working with the legs turned out can improve this muscle tone. With legs held parallel it is harder to overrecruit the gluteus maximus, nor can we pinch our buttocks together as easily, thus the abdominals work better. Also, with parallel feet the internal rotators will not lock as easily in an attempt to counteract the force of the powerful external rotators.

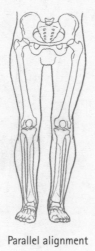

Parallel alignment

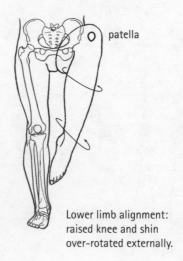

patella

Lower limb alignment: raised knee and shin over-rotated externally.

Lower limb alignment

In parallel alignment the second toe is in line with the middle of the kneecap (or patella) and the kneecap is in line with the middle of the front of the hip, in both the lengthened, softly pointed position or the dorsiflexed (toes to shin) position.

In the turned-out position the whole leg should still be in this alignment, just externally rotated. This recruits the large, most superficial buttock muscle, the gluteus maximus.

However, when the leg is bent at the knee the lower limb can rotate out still further, leading to mis-alignment through the leg. With a bent knee the badly controlled shin and foot can turn out another twenty degrees, even when the knee and thigh remain parallel. If the legs are straightened with the lower leg still turned out the knee can be strained. Thus in work which involves bending and straightening the leg, keep the whole leg in alignment, including the shin, ankle and foot.

Poor alignment of legs and feet is often a problem for dancers, and can lead to serious faults in technique that cause both knee and ankle problems. It can also be a problem for runners, and in any sport such as netball where running and sudden stops and twists are inherent in the sport.

SINGLE LEG STRETCH BASED ON KNEE FLOAT ACTION

Aim:

To encourage the abdominals to work more strongly. This is an original Pilates exercise that was primarily a leg, arm and chest exercise but has been modified in modern Pilates to encourage the abdominals to work more. The height of the leg extension is regulated by your ability to keep the centre of your body in neutral and to hold it there.

To start, lie on your back with both legs bent, raised off the floor with the knees slightly toward the waist, lower legs parallel to the floor, toes lengthened away.

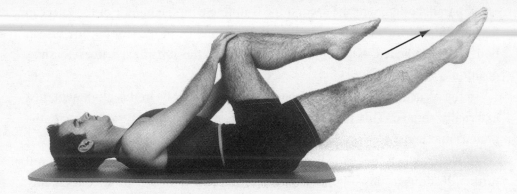

Rest your hands lightly on your knees and keep your head relaxed on the floor.

Inhale and connect with your centre. Begin to exhale, flattening and narrowing your stomach and engaging all your abdominal muscles. Extend one leg away from your body at about 45 degrees, ensuring the abdominals continue to support the spine as your leg stretches. Your spine remains in a neutral position, gently resting on the floor. Place both hands lightly on the other knee. Inhale as you bend the straightened leg back in to its original position. Ensure that your spine remains relaxed on the floor. Repeat with the other leg, exhaling as you straighten it and support your centre. Place both hands on the bent knee.

Repeat 6 times on each side. As you get stronger increase to 10 times each side.

Visualisation:

You are reaching away with your foot to the far wall, in a long line from the centre.

Points of caution:

Take care not to speed up your breathing or to bend the bent leg further in toward your chest—this will cause it to act as a counterbalance and thus reduce the work of your centre. It is important to coordinate your leg movements with your breath flow. The further you lengthen your leg away from your body the harder it is to hold your abdominals down and keep your spine in neutral, so only stretch your leg to the point where your centre is still in control of the leg movement, always maintaining good leg alignment.

Variations:

As you get stronger and more stable you can increase the difficulty of the exercise by elevating the upper body and head (this is similar to the original version). In some ways this makes the exercise easier because the work of lifting the head and shoulders recruits the upper chest muscles (pectoralis major) and intercostals to help. Make sure all the work still comes from the centre.

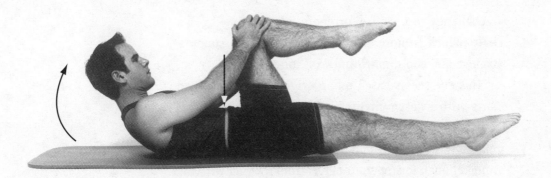

Points of caution:

Take extra care not to strongly grasp the leg with the hands and pull it toward the shoulder; this makes the arm and chest muscles work too hard. It is important to curve through the spine and lift from under the shoulders. Ensure that the front of the hip lengthens with a released joint and reach out with the leg. Do not just force the leg to straighten.

Advanced variations:

Interlock the hands behind the head and twist the upper body, reaching diagonally across the chest with the opposite elbow toward the bent knee; keep the elbows open, and pull back the elbow nearest the floor. You can also change the breathing pattern to inhale on the leg stretch and exhale as the other leg stretches, to increase the speed.

Do not attempt these variations if you have a neck problem.

SINGLE LEG CIRCLES

Aim:

To challenge your centre further by moving one leg in a circle (which is more difficult for the body to support, stabilise and coordinate) and working the legs.

This exercise is based on an original exercise which starts with a large circular movement. You will start with a small circle with the leg slightly bent, only enlarging the circle when your abdominal muscles are strong enough to stop your pelvis from rocking with the leg movement.

To start, lie in constructive rest position and raise one leg toward the ceiling, knee bent, toes softly pointed, while keeping the pelvis and spine aligned on the floor, arms resting by your side. Extend your lower leg along the floor and straighten the lifted leg. Both

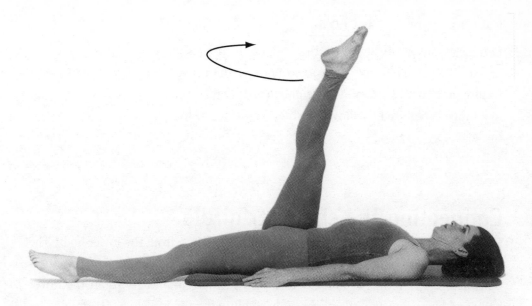

hips must remain on the floor. If you are unable to straighten the raised leg without lifting your hip, you can keep the lifted leg slightly bent.

Inhale. As you exhale trace a circular shape with the raised leg going across the body first, then back down toward the floor and slightly outward, completing the circle by bringing your leg up toward the ceiling. Inhale as your leg comes up. Continue the circle, exhaling as your leg moves around and away from the body.

Repeat the circle 4 times in the same direction, then circle 4 times the other way. Change legs, circling 4 times with the leg going across the body and 4 times in the outwards direction. As you get stronger increase the repetitions to 6 in both directions.

Visualisation:

You are drawing a large letter O on the ceiling with your toe, with your leg following a smooth, swooping motion.

Points of caution:

Extra care needs to be taken that only the lifted leg
moves. Do not move the leg on the floor or the torso.
Ensure that your centre remains stable. Good hamstring
flexibility is required to allow the lifted leg to reach for
the ceiling.

26 Connecting the shoulder girdle

The upper body and arms have a very different function from the lower body. The
upper body needs to be able to help the hands grasp and reach and has the potential for a bigger range of movements, with greater complexity, than the lower
body and legs. However, the upper body's ability to move freely is determined by
the strength and balance of the lower body and the centre. The ribcage is supported by the abdominal muscles. Between each rib the intercostal muscles travel
in pathways similar to the oblique abdominals. There is a muscular connection
from the centre to the shoulders via the external oblique abdominal, which interdigitates with the serratus anterior. So how well the shoulders work relates to how
the ribs, the thoracic spine and abdominals function. Arm movement is affected
by shoulder alignment and support (which is technically referred to as the
humero-scapular rhythm).

Lumbar protection and thoracic extension

I suggest you revise the information on the shoulder and arm on pages 78–80.
Once you have comfortably achieved the elbow lift and the diamond press in the
basic programme you can continue with stabilising your shoulder and further
challenging your lower and mid back while protecting the lower back. This more
complex work is aimed at connecting the shoulder region with the whole body
via the lateral diagonal muscles of the body, with the spine sustaining good
alignment.

The spine has gentle curves both forward and backward. The depth and form
of these curves are unique to each of us. Where a curve becomes exaggerated

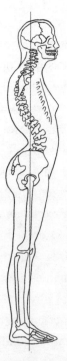

Shortened lordosis, lengthened kyphosis

long-term problems can result. The kyphosis of the thoracic region frequently starts too low, which not only puts pressure on the lordosis of the lumbar spine, but also reduces the ability of the lower thorax to extend. Thus when we bend backward (extend) we are mostly using the lower back or lumbar spine, while the mid back, or lower thoracic region, where the lower ribs attach to the spine, tends to stay either flat or in a fixed curve forwards (a slight kyphosis). This poor posture can be made worse by performing abdominal crunches with the head pulled up, and by any overuse of the upper abdominals and chest muscles (pectorals) with resistance work, such as may occur in medicine ball workouts. Because the upper abdominals are easier to connect with we tend to scrunch them in, which compresses the lower ribcage back into the spine and further increases the kyphosis (see p. 120).

Modern Pilates recognises that we need to be able to work and hold the lower abdominals while stretching the upper abdominals so that flexibility in the mid spine is sustained over a lifetime. Many important muscles attach to the mid spine, such as the crus of the diaphragm, the psoas, the serratus posterior inferior, the quadratus lumborum, the superficial and deep erector spinae (multifidus) and part of the broad back muscle (latissimus dorsi). Thus this area has a lot of muscles potentially putting pressure on the region.

The area of the mid back is hard to see, touch and sense. It's the bit we slump into the back of a chair and begin to curve forward in poor posture. It is a transition area in terms of bony structure and soft tissue. The direct relationship with the diaphragm firmly connects the mid back with breathing and the effects breathing has on the display and experience of emotion. Whether we are laughing, crying, shouting in rage or excitement, or controlling the expression of emotion, this area is moved, held or stretched in response. We store and contain much emotional expression in this area. This region, the mid to lower thoracic, is the centre or middle of the body in babies and children. It is only when we grow to full height and our legs lengthen at physical maturity that the centre lowers to include the lower pelvis. (Do we sometimes get stuck in a childlike posture?)

How the base of the ribcage is supported affects the whole of the upper body and the carriage of the head. It affects how we feel about ourselves. Working through the next exercises will improve your upper body alignment and help prevent the acquisition of a 'widow's hump' (sometimes called a 'dowager's hump').

SPHINX TO SINGLE LEG FLICK

Aim:

To increase mid back or lower thoracic extension while protecting the lumbar spine and keeping shoulder alignment.

To start, lie on your stomach (prone) with legs softly together and toes lengthened. Place your arms, bent at the elbow, next to your body with palms to the floor and hands on the floor near your shoulders.

Inhale. As you exhale, support your centre by lifting the lower abdomen up, then press down on forearms

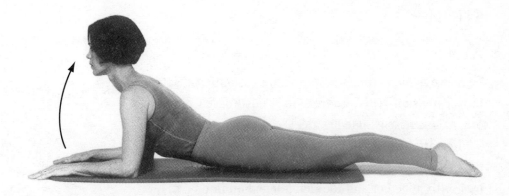

and hands, lifting the upper body and head up off the mat. Stretch the upper abdomen and curve the mid spine into extension, opening the chest. Inhale as you lower your body back to the mat to the start position.

Repeat 6 times.

Visualisation:

You are lifting your chest up like the prow of a ship, lengthening your upper chest, sternum and head away from the hips, so that you look like the sphinx in Egypt.

Points of caution:

Take care not to let the lower abdominals relax. Do not push down into the lower spine and overextend the lower back. Make sure that the upper abdominals are lengthened.

Variation:

If you are comfortable in the sphinx position and can continue to use the abdominals to support the lower back, stay with the upper body lifted, resting on the forearms, and add a leg bend and stretch that becomes a single leg flick.

SINGLE LEG FLICK

Aim:

To improve hamstring strength while sustaining a safe back extension. This progression is also based on an original exercise (single leg kick).

To start, lie in sphinx position with the forearms on the floor and the upper body extended up off the floor, legs softly together and toes lengthened on floor.

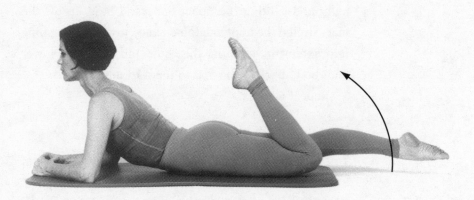

Inhale as you bend one leg to reach your foot towards your buttock with a gentle flicking motion, then exhale and stretch the leg out straight, slightly off the floor. As you straighten the leg, press down on elbows and forearms and lengthen your upper body, supporting the lower abdomen up and protecting the lower spine. Inhale, soften the body and repeat the leg flick on the other side. Keep the toes softly pointed.

Repeat 8 times each side, alternating legs.

Visualisation:

You are reaching your heel to buttock as though the leg is a rubber band. As you straighten the leg imagine you are reaching the top of your head toward the ceiling.

Points of caution:

Take care to not collapse your body to the floor as you bend the leg. Ensure that you lift your lower abdomen while supporting your lower back as you extend the leg. Do not do this exercise if you have sore knees or any discomfort in your lower back.

PLANK

Aim:

To improve the balance and strength of front and back muscles, with cross-diagonal support. This is a strength exercise using the hip flexors lengthened. This challenges the shoulder stabilising muscles and abdominals to support the back strongly and keep good postural alignment.

To start, take up the 4-point kneeling position with the arms very slightly bent, shoulder-width apart. Inhale. Reach one leg back and place the ball of your foot on the floor, fully extending the leg and placing your weight on it. As you exhale, extend the other leg back in a straight line so that you put your weight on both the balls of the feet evenly. The body forms a straight line between shoulders and heels. Hold this position for four breaths. Then bend the legs in and down to the floor, one at a time, to go back to 4-point kneeling.

Repeat 4 times.

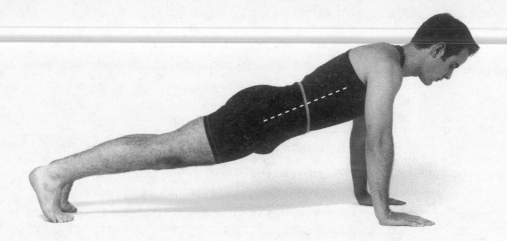

Visualisation:

Your head is reaching away from your feet as if you are a rocket.

Points of caution:

Take care not to sag at the waist or to tuck your pelvis under. Do not overuse your buttock muscles. Ensure your arms and shoulders are supported with the spine in neutral alignment.

Modification:

Rest on your forearms if your wrists are uncomfortable taking weight.

27 Articulating the spine

The spine is a series of 24 small, similarly-shaped complex bones (the vertebrae) plus the sacrum and coccyx. It's a bit like a tower of hats with triangular holey brims sitting on an upside-down pyramid. The bones of the spine help support the torso and protect the spinal cord, from which the main nerves pass to the rest of the body, and most importantly allows us to make complex multi-directional movements. A flexible spine lets us twist, turn and spiral in many different ways.

Joe Pilates thought that the spine should be flat (see Chapter 1) and absolutely straight. Present-day Pilates method teaches respect for the natural curves of the spine and has modified the traditional Pilates exercises so they are done in a supported neutral spine position. Pilates was correct, however, in understanding that having a flexible spine is important for movement ability and that stretching, articulating and strengthening the spine would help to improve posture.

The spine is made up of alternating hard, complex-shaped bony vertebrae and cushioning pillows of intervertebral disc that are squashed by gravity during the day. Each vertebra is connected to the next by two pairs of facet joints and some very strong ligaments, that permit a variable range of movement.

The structure of the spine

The back of the pelvis is made up of a triangular bone called the sacrum, with a small tail of 2–4 vertebrae called the coccyx. The base of the spine is embedded in and very strongly bound to the large wing bones of the pelvis via the sacrum, which is made up of five fused vertebrae. The five lumbar vertebrae sit on top, with powerful ligaments supporting the relatively rigid sacrum and connecting to the moveable lumbar vertebrae.

The lumbar spine is made up of five large vertebrae and has good forward and backward flexibility but relatively limited spiral movement. Above the lumbar spine is the thoracic spine (12 vertebrae) with the ribs attached to the sides of the vertebrae. The thoracic vertebrae are more tightly bound than the lumbar verte-brae, having less forward and backward movement but the potential for more spiral movement.

Above the thoracic vertebrae is the cervical spine (the neck). The seven cervical vertebrae are much more delicate than the other vertebrae, and are the most flexible group. They can bend forward and back as well as spirally and tilt laterally, with the top two vertebrae working together to allow the head to pivot freely through a large range of movement.

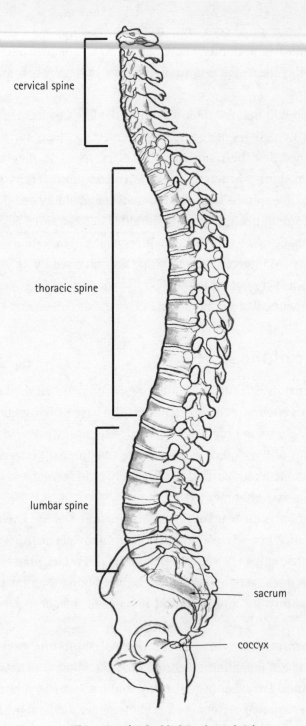

cervical spine

thoracic spine

lumbar spine

sacrum

coccyx

The spine (embedded in the pelvis)

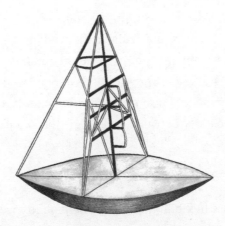

The spine has a mast, anchored by the muscular guyropes (after Weineck)

Many slender muscles link the vertebrae for support and to allow movement. The spine is held together with layers of ligaments, tendons and muscles. At the back, the deeper posterior muscles (deep erector spinae—multifidus) tend to be shorter, linking small groups of vertebrae together. The more superficial erector spinae muscles tend to be longer, acting over many vertebrae. There are very few muscles along the front (inside) of the spine travelling directly up and down (except for the psoas major and minor which attach to the 12th thoracic vertebrae and all the lumbar vertebrae before travelling down to the femur). But many muscles are attached to the sides of the spine, wrapping around toward the front of the torso. The spine is a bit like the mast of a sailing boat anchored into the pelvis (the hull of the boat), with guy ropes of muscles supporting it.

Gravity acts directly on the spine, compressing the spaces between the vertebrae during the day. This is why we are shorter in the evening than we are when we get out of bed in the morning. Gravity tends to compress the lumbar spine backwards and down, increasing its natural lordosis. The ribs then press down onto the abdomen as the thoracic spine curves forwards and down in kyphosis. Any specific weakness in the muscles of the torso, such as weak oblique abdominals, can also strongly affect the alignment of the spine.

Improving the articulation and flexibility of the spine has to be done with a strong awareness of what parts of it are over-flexible and vulnerable, and what areas are held rigid. We must aim to support the flexible parts with focused awareness and only stretch the groups of tight vertebrae in ways that will not overstretch the mobile areas. Particular care needs to be taken in some specific areas. The commonly over-mobile areas are at the base of the spine, from the lower two lumbar vertebrae to the sacrum. We need to use the oblique abdominals to protect and support these areas. The commonly over-tight region is the thoracic spine, particularly between and below the shoulder blades.

The spine and hamstrings

To improve the spine's flexibility and movement ability we need to stretch it carefully, and support it with the wrap-around stomach muscles, including the oblique abdominals. Stretching and moving the spine affects the pelvis and leg muscles. Care needs to be taken when mobilising the spine because the length of the leg muscles can affect spinal movement.

Very short hamstrings commonly contribute to lower back problems, as the hamstrings hold the lower part of the pelvis and hence affect the lower spine. When there is no flexibility in the hamstrings they do not release the pelvis to allow forward movement of the body. When this happens only the spine bends, placing huge strain and stress on the lower back. If the pelvis is held upright by short hamstrings, as you straighten up from a forward bend only the lower back muscles and buttock muscle can work to draw the body upright, which increases the effort and the compression in the lower back. Thus it is very important to have flexible hamstrings.

How to check on hamstring length

The hamstrings attach to the base of the pelvis at the sitting bones and travel down the thigh to the back of the knees, at the sides. If you bend forward and reach for the floor from standing with legs straight, or sit on the floor with legs out in front and reach forward, you will be able to tell how flexible your hamstrings are and how much flexing or bending forward your back does. However, both these movements can cause back strain and should not be done if you have any sort of back problem.

The safe way to check for hamstring flexibility is to lie on the floor and stretch and straighten one leg at a time up to the ceiling, carefully keeping the back on the floor and the pelvis in neutral. This ensures that the back does not bend and the pelvis does not tuck under or tilt.

Done along with the kneeling hamstring stretch from the basic programme, this next exercise will increase hamstring flexibility. I cannot stress enough that good hamstring flexibility is vital for getting on with ordinary life comfortably. We should all have hamstrings long enough to be able to release the pelvis forward when we bend over or, as in this next exercise, be able to reach the raised leg to the ceiling.

SUPINE HAMSTRING STRETCH WITH A TOWEL OR BELT

Aim:

To improve hamstring flexibility through active resisted movement.

To start, lie on your back in constructive rest position. Raise one leg and place the middle of a towel or a belt under the arch of your foot. Hold the ends of the towel one in each hand.

Inhale and align your spine, ensuring that the base of your spine and tail bone are firmly on the mat. As you exhale, lengthen the raised leg towards the ceiling, using the towel to help support the leg as it extends, at the same time keeping the pelvis in neutral. Inhale and pause with the leg extended, then exhale and, holding the towel firmly, try to stretch the leg downward while resisting the movement with the arms holding the towel still. Inhale and draw the leg toward your body by bending your arms, keeping the leg straight. Exhale, and relax the leg down towards the floor.

Repeat 5 times on each side, using slow movements.

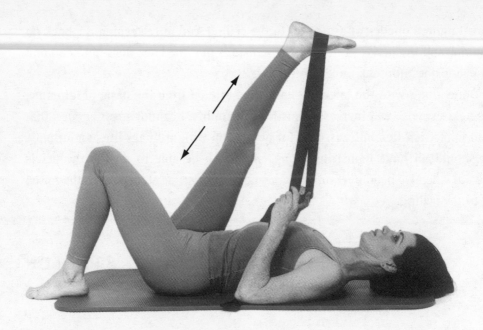

Visualisation:

An equal amount of lengthening at the top of the leg near the buttocks down into the floor and as well as at the heel reaching up to the ceiling.

Points of caution:

Take care not to press the lower back into the floor or tilt the pelvis. Do not get carried away trying to pull your leg to your body, thus allowing the spine to distort. Do not place the towel on the ball of the foot, as this will increase the stretch by putting strain on the calf.

Stretching the spine

Normally the exercises in this group are done on the floor, but to avoid lower back problems or over-challenging hamstring flexibility at first, sit on a dining chair or kitchen chair with your feet firmly on the ground. Done completely upright on a chair, these spine stretches primarily challenge the spine's flexibility. Stretching the spine while sitting on the floor also challenges the flexibility of the hamstrings.

The variation you choose is dependent on the flexibility of the backs of the legs. If you have short hamstrings, practise the versions sitting on a chair. Also practise the kneeling hamstring stretch from the basic programme, every day, to improve hamstring flexibility.

SEATED SPINE STRETCH

Aim:

To articulate or move the spine through each vertebra evenly, without over-stretching any spinal joint or holding any areas tight.

To start, inhale, sitting up tall, on a chair in neutral spine. As you exhale, curl down from the top of the head, slowly curving the spine one vertebra at a time towards the floor. Relax the arms down by the sides of the legs. Keep drawing in the stomach. Inhale when you reach maximum curlover and relax. Start to exhale, uncurling from the base of the spine up to the start position.

Repeat 8 times.

Visualisation:

You are curling over a large beach ball and cannot collapse the front of the body as you lengthen out the back of the spine.

Points of caution:

Take care not to roll back onto your buttocks, but stay upright on your seat bones.

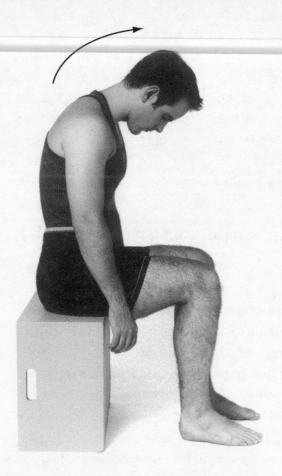

Variation:

As your ability to articulate through your spine improves, curl and uncurl on a single breath cycle, inhaling on the way up.

SPINE STRETCH

Aim:

To articulate through the spine while supporting your centre with lengthening hamstrings.

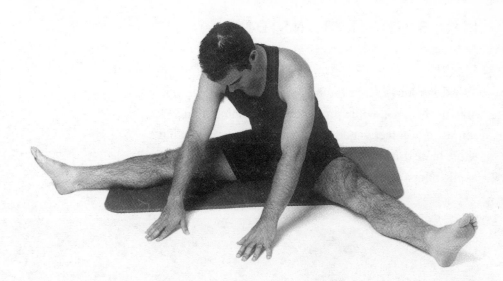

To start, sit on a pillow on the floor, with your legs stretched out, as far apart as is comfortable, fingertips just off the floor between your parted legs, feet relaxed.

Inhale, sitting up tall. As you exhale, curl down through your spine, reaching forward with the fingers as far away as possible from your body and narrowing your waist as you curl down through the spine one vertebra at a time. Keep your lower abdominals working. Inhale as you uncurl and return to the upright position.

Repeat 6 to 8 times.

Visualisation:

Reach forward beyond the toes and at the same time reach down through the tailbone, as though your spine is a willow tree curving down with the roots firmly anchored in the ground through your sitting bones.

Points of caution:

Take care to keep the sitting bones firmly on the floor throughout the whole movement and return the torso to an aligned upright position. Do not tilt or lean forward.

MID SPINE EXTENSION

Aim:

To extend and stretch the mid spine, the lower thoracic area of the back, while protecting the lumbar spine. Use the sitting on feet version at first, especially if you have short hamstrings, moving on to the knees bent version as the hamstrings lengthen.

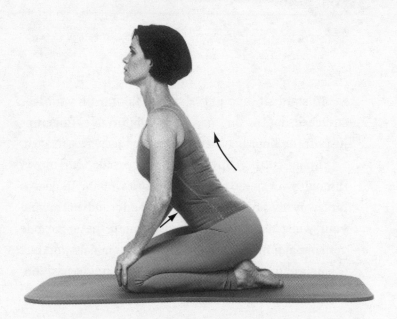

To start, bend your legs underneath you and sit on your feet (you may need a pillow between your feet and your bottom). Place one hand on each knee (you will have to lean forward slightly to do this) so your body is at a slight forward angle.

Inhale and soften the spine into a slight curve inward, relaxing the head down. Start to exhale, connecting with your centre and pressing down on your hands to help lift the mid to upper body out and up towards the ceiling. The sternum lifts away from the waist, stretching the mid back into slight extension.

The hands and arms help to create traction by working with the elbows held slightly bent and out toward the side. This helps to separate the vertebrae, lengthening your spine as you work.

Repeat 4 times.

Visualisation:

Your upper body and neck become long and elegant, like the neck of a swan, as you lift your sternum upward.

Points of caution:

Take care to focus on the centre, and not to over arch the lower back forward so that you do not let go of the lower abdominals. Ensure that your ribs do not stick out.

Modification:

When you are able to do this sitting on your feet, and your hamstrings have lengthened and the fronts of your hip are relaxed, sit on the floor with knees bent and feet flat on the floor, with your body upright on your sitting bones. Hold your knees gently with each hand.

Inhale. As you exhale hold knees firmly, draw your chest slightly towards your knees and lift your chest to the ceiling.

Variation:

Try lifting one arm up to the ceiling as you stretch your back out. Reach forward and upward with the hand, lifting the arm overhead as you extend your mid back.

So far we have stretched and articulated the spine without changing the overall balance or increasing weightbearing.

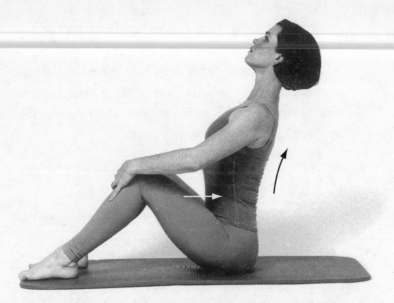

Add this next exercise only after you are very comfortable with the previous stretches and can feel an even articulation throughout your spine with no discomfort.

ROLLING

Aim:

To massage the spine and load it throughout its articulation, while improving awareness of body weight, balance and the impact of momentum. If you have any area of rigidity or discomfort in your spine do not attempt this exercise (this is a modified original exercise).

To start, sit on the mat with the legs bent, with your knees fairly close to your chest. Wrap your arms around your legs, lightly resting one hand on the other in front of your shins.

Inhale with the head softly bent forward, then exhale and connect with your centre. Inhale, and roll back through your spine until you are resting on your

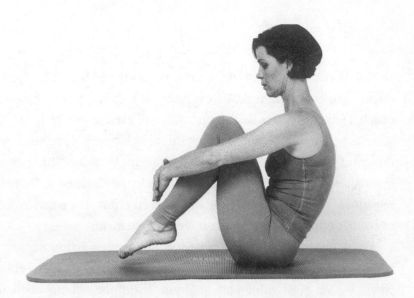

shoulders, still in a curved ball shape. Exhale, and roll back through the spine to sitting, using your abdominals to bring you back to the upright position.

Repeat 6 times.

Visualisation:

You are a large beach ball rolling gently backward and forward, up and down the beach as the waves break.

Points of caution:

Take care to control the rolling. Do not use too much momentum, do not pull with your arms. Keep your hands slightly away from your shins. Try to use your abdominals to keep the round shape. Ensure that your head does not hit the floor on the roll back.

Variation:

When you are comfortable with this, try keeping your feet softly lengthened and off the floor the whole time and balancing on your bottom in the upright position.

28 Spirals

The spine can move in all directions. Forward and back are the simplest move-ments—but the least-used in everyday life. Straight movements are usually coupled with a spiral twist and turn or bend, even if only to facilitate reaching for something in the cupboard, turning on the ignition, putting the key in the lock of the front door. Spiralling is a vital movement ability, directly related to the crossed extensor reflex which is active in all balance activities and upright movement. There is a criss-cross of balanced effort. The waist is the crossroads of one side's effort against the other side's movement.

Moving in spirals is the most common complex action that our body does. It is the last movement ability we learn to support or stabilise as children. It is also where we are most vulnerable to strain. Using the oblique abdominals with the deeper transversus abdominis to lengthen the waist as we spiral is vitally impor-tant to help protect the lower back from strain.

These next exercises challenge your ability to twist or spiral the spine and improve its flexibility.

THE SAW

Aim:

To improve the spine's spiral flexibility (original exercise).

If you have very short hamstrings this exercise can be done on a chair the same way as spine stretch. With moderately short hamstrings sit on pillows on the floor.

To start, sit up, with the body tall and perpendicular to the floor, the legs stretched out wide apart, toes lifted to the ceiling. Lift your arms up and out to the sides at shoulder height, with palms to the floor.

Inhale. As you exhale spiral the body around towards one leg, reaching forward with the opposite arm and moving the body across the leg. Extend this

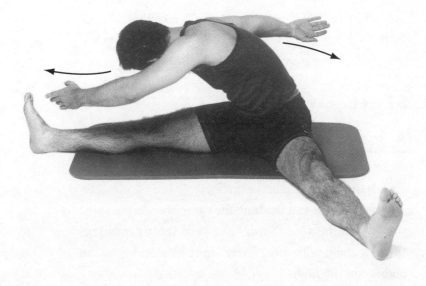

arm towards the little-toe side of the foot, with the palm of the hand facing away from the foot. At the same time as twisting your spine, lengthen your body downward so that the little finger is reaching for the little toe and the opposite hip is working to ensure the hips stay squarely on the floor. Open the back arm out and extend the spiral so the head is looking round towards this hand, behind you. Inhale and return to the upright position with the arms still out to the side.

Repeat 3 to 5 times alternating sides.

Visualisation:

You are reaching up and away with the top of the head, spiralling gracefully through the spine, as though you are slowly twisting the top off a bottle.

Points of caution:

Take care to keep the centre firmly anchored, with the sitting bones connected to the floor. Ensure that the legs stay still with the knees pointing to the ceiling. Do not let the leg that you are working away from roll inward.

SPINE TWIST

Aim:

To improve the ability of the thorax to spiral and to stretch the spine (original exercise).

This exercise can be done the same way as the spine stretch and the saw: if you have very short hamstrings sit on a chair, with moderately short hamstrings sit on pillows on the floor.

To start, sit up tall, with your body at right angles to the floor, your legs extended forward and the inner sides of your feet touching, toes softly pointed. Reach your arms out to the side at shoulder height, lengthen your arms, palms down, elbows in line with your shoulders, to take tension away from neck.

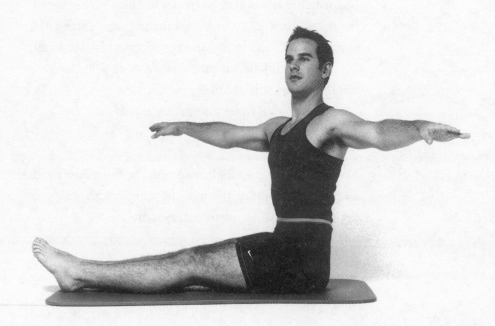

Inhale. As you exhale spiral your body around to one side as you lengthen your head to the ceiling. With further effort on the last of the exhale, try to increase stretch and spiral further. Inhale as you return to start position.

Repeat 3 to 5 times each side.

Visualisation:

Your body is a screwtop jar; you try to twist off the top as you move.

Variation:

If you have neck or shoulder tension bend your arms up so that your fingertips rest on your shoulders.

Points of caution:

Take care to spiral only through the body, ensuring that the arms do not bend at the shoulders. Do not bounce or force this stretch. Lengthen your spine as you spiral.

29 Diagonal and lateral connections

We often ignore the sides of our bodies, tending to think only in terms of front and back, and forgetting the bit in the middle, the depth through the body.

We are three-dimensional, with muscles that connect front and back tending to curve around in arcs or parts of spirals in our bodies. The inside and outside leg and hip muscles also perform an important role, controlling lateral sway. When we stand and walk they work in conjunction with our side abdominal muscles to stop us from wobbling from side to side.

Focusing on these lateral connections is easier if you lie on your side. Gravity helps to create resistance, thus increasing your awareness of the parts of the body resting on the floor and those working directly against gravity.

Bracing is not centring

A brace is a rigid support with fixed struts or stays. Abdominal bracing, much used in traditional Pilates and some other exercise prescriptions, is very carefully avoided in modern Pilates as rigidity is anathema to the method. Modern Pilates concentrates on centring. It is easiest to see the difference between bracing and centring when you are exercising lying on your side. In bracing, the body is compressed with intraabdominal pressure, usually applied via held inspiration with the upper body fixed. It is an action rarely needed in everyday life—only for urgent heavy lifting or occasionally when one is constipated. When bracing is used in the side lie position the waist is unable to be lifted and narrowed. When a load is placed on the braced area, such as when the legs lift sideways, the hips move towards the ribs as the pressure of the bracing pushes the lower side of the body into the floor, over-recruiting the buttocks and adductors. Being able to feel gentle abdominal movement during breathing means that the trunk is not braced, but is centred.

Once you have achieved side breathing and clams from the basic programme you can add these next side lie exercises to your workout.

SIDE DOUBLE LEG LIFT

Aim:

To increase awareness and connection with the sides of the body, improve side abdominal strength and lateral support, and start building inside and outside hip and leg strength.

To start, lie on your side, stretched out as straight as possible, toes lengthened away from you, with your head resting on the underneath arm, your legs resting one on top of the other, feet together. Use the top arm to help you balance, placing your hand on the floor in front of your chest.

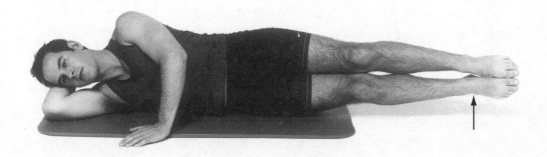

Inhale. As you exhale narrow the waist, connect with your centre and support the hips. Lift the top leg up to be parallel with the floor, then bring the lower leg up to touch along the length of the top leg without tilting or twisting the pelvis. Your lateral abdominals will be working strongly. Inhale and lower both legs to the floor, slowly and evenly.

Repeat 8 times each side.

Visualisation:

Reach the legs away from the centre of the body as though someone is pulling them to the opposite wall.

Points of caution:

Take care to keep the hips lengthened away from the ribs with the pelvis in alignment. Do not overuse the upper body or press hard on the front arm.

SIDE LEG SWING (KICK)

Aim:

To connect the spirals of the body and practise contra-lateral movement as the leg swings forward and back, stabilising side torso strength (modified original exercise).

To start, lie in the side lie position, with the head off the floor, supported in line with the spine by the lower hand, fingers resting at the back of the head. The upper arm is bent with the hand resting lightly on the floor in front of the chest. The legs are together and extended slightly forward from the body. Inhale. Bring the top leg straight forward, parallel to the floor and towards your chest with the foot flexed up. As you exhale, steadily swing the upper leg straight back, toes lengthened. As the leg moves behind your body ensure that you lengthen and lift the waist using the obliques. Reach the leg behind you as far as you can without letting go of your centre. Inhale. Soften the side of the body down on the floor as you repeat the forward swing with the foot flexed up.

Repeat 8 times on one side, then roll over onto the other hip and repeat 8 times.

Visualisation:

Your leg swings freely like a pendulum.

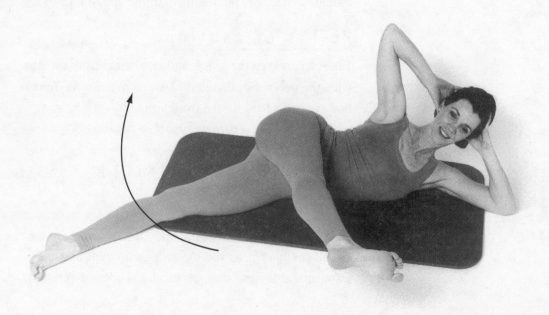

Points of caution:

Take care not to move the lower leg. Keep the pelvis at a right angle to floor.

Variations:

When you are comfortable with this version reduce your upper body support by bending both arms at the elbows and placing both hands behind the head. You are now resting only on the elbow of the arm nearest the floor. As you swing your leg back on exhalation, remember to elevate the body off the floor by using your obliques and the muscles under your armpits. Your elbow, hips and lower leg remain on the floor.

30 Lower pelvic stabilisers

Pilates method exercises, at any level from basic to advanced, differ greatly from many other forms of exercise in that there is no impact through the body. When we jog, run, go to the gym, jump, or lift heavy weights in the upright position, we jar the body and put pressure down into the pelvis. Jumping up and down causes the contents of our torso to bounce down with the help of gravity and press into the lower pelvis or pelvic floor. When this happens many kilograms of weight push down onto the pelvis and impact on our pelvic floor muscles. Those muscles help with reproduction (with gender specific variations), allow outflow from the digestive system, control when we go to the toilet, and are the prime site of sexual excitement. They also help with external rotation and abduction of the thigh and connect with the abdominal muscles. Thus the pelvic floor is a very important area to keep toned and connected.

The pelvic floor and the centre

The traditional Pilates centre, located between the lower ribs and a line across the top of the hips, completely ignored the pelvic floor. The muscles of the pelvic floor are very relevant to modern Pilates, however, as they make up the lower border of the newly defined centre and support pelvic stabilisation. They also interact with the thoracic diaphragm. The pelvic floor is just like any other area of the body—if it is weak, or overbraced, it will not function well, which can cause many problems so, it needs to be exercised.

The muscles of the lower pelvis are made up of the pelvic wall and pelvic floor. Numerous muscles and ligaments form a complex hammock that stops the viscera drooping to the floor. The physiology and anatomy of the pelvic floor muscles are firmly connected to the rest of the abdominal region. The oblique abdominal muscles wrap around and help create the inguinal canal, which is under the slender diagonal band at the base of the abdomen that forms the crease between the leg and the torso. The lower part of the internal oblique curves up and out, and the lower part of the external oblique curls down and in to enfold the inguinal ligament. The covering of the superficial inguinal ring encloses the spermatic cord and cremaster muscle in men, and the round ligament that holds up the uterus in women.

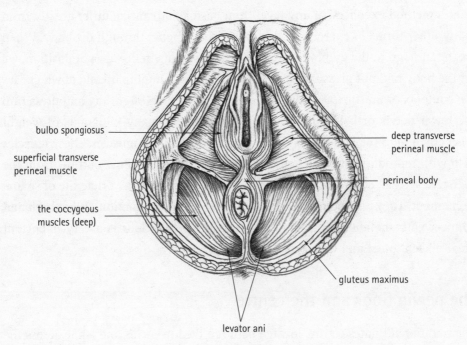

The pelvic floor (after Platzer)

Finding your pelvic floor

Following the diagram you can see that the pelvic floor is made up of a number of muscles surrounding the lower outlets of the body—the urethra and vagina (or penis and testes) in front and the anus to the rear, surrounded by a band of muscle in the shape of a figure '8', all of which make up the perineum.

Simply tightening the outside muscles of the pelvic floor may only marginally reduce incontinence, as part of the problem may be due to the viscera pressing downward on to the bladder. It is important to imagine the interior muscles that support the pelvic bowl and be careful not to confuse the large buttock and thigh muscles with the pelvic floor. Two external rotators deep in the buttocks do contribute to the make-up of the pelvic wall, but squeezing the buttocks and legs together will not necessarily engage them.

SINGLE PELVIC LIFTS FOR MEN AND WOMEN

Aim:

To strengthen the pelvic floor muscles.

To start, lie in a supported or constructive rest position. Inhale firmly downwards, feeling the abdomen expand. Sense the pelvic floor, particularly at the perineum, gently bulge outwards and relax. Exhale and lift the pelvic floor, drawing up towards the middle of the body. As the pelvic floor lifts, connect with the lower abdominal muscles, particularly the pyramidalis, which lies just above the pubic bone. This is the most important lowest part of breathing. When it is working well there is a slight rolling of the pelvis and hips.

LIFT AND HOLD FOR WOMEN— (THE ELEVATOR)

Aim:

To strengthen the vaginal muscles.

This next exercise is a follow-along visualisation. Imagine the vagina is a lift shaft with a smoothly running elevator in a building with three floors. This exercise will improve subtle muscle engagement.

- The ground floor is the natural relaxed position at the surface opening of the vagina.

- The next floor is the middle of the vagina.

- The top floor is the top of the vagina where the cervix lies.

Inhale, and imagine the elevator is resting poised at the ground floor and the doors are opening to let a passenger in. The passenger presses the buttons to close the doors as you exhale; continue to exhale as the lift rises to take them to the next floor. Hold the exhale as the passenger gets out of the lift. Inhale, as more people get into the lift (hold the lift steady as you inhale). These passengers wish to go to the top floor. Exhale as the lift travels to the top floor, hold the lift as the people get out, and inhale. (This next bit is the hardest.) Exhale as the lift is lowered to the middle floor, hold the lift steady as passengers get in, inhale. These people wish to go to the ground floor. Exhale as the lift lowers to the ground, inhale as you let the passengers out, relax.

Repeat this exercise 1 to 3 times a day.

ELEVATOR FOR MEN

Aim:

To improve the connection between male pelvic floor muscles.

Inhale. Feel the perineum bulge very slightly. As you exhale, lift and tighten the ring of muscle surrounding the penis and running behind the scrotum as though you are gripping a ball. This will elevate the penis slightly. Hold the feeling of lifting and gripping as you finish the exhale, then inhale and continue with the lifting sensation, exhale and try to lift the muscles of the perineum higher. Inhale to partially let go the feeling of gripping, as though you are slightly loosening your hold on a ball. Exhale and continue to hold gently. Then inhale, completely let go and relax the pelvic floor fully on the exhale.

Repeat 6 times.

Points of caution (both women and men):

Take care not to use the quadriceps, buttocks or inside thighs or tilt the pelvis up. When things are not working well the pelvic floor muscles are slack and unresponsive, like a lift flopped into the basement with loose cables, or jammed just above ground floor. As the pelvic floor begins to work better you may have feelings of warmth, or some internal muscle soreness. It is very important never to overdo pelvic floor exercises—these muscles can fatigue and strain and too easily recruit other, inappropriate muscles. Awareness, precision and lots of persistence over time are required to achieve lasting change.

Inside thighs

The inside thighs also help to stabilise the pelvis and hold the legs together. If we often sit for long periods of time (as at a computer-based job) the inside thighs tend to lock into a holding pattern of minimal effort and short range. It is important to increase their strength, as well as to stretch them. It is also important to distinguish them from the pelvic floor muscles.

PILLOW SQUEEZE

Aim:

To improve and work the adductor muscles for inside thigh strength.

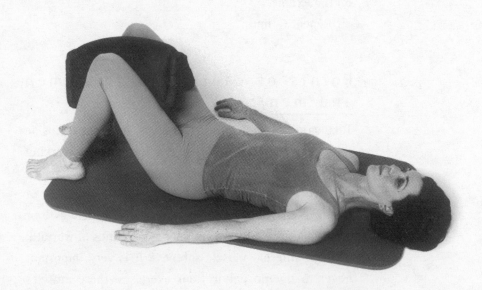

To start, lie in the constructive rest position, with your legs hip-width apart. Place a couple of firm pillows between your knees.

Inhale. As you exhale draw the insides of the knees toward each other, compressing the pillows, then relax the legs apart as you inhale.

Repeat for 6 slow squeezes.

Visualisation:

The upper hips and back of the pelvis are spreading and relaxing apart as you press the insides of your knees together.

Points of caution:

Take care not to tuck and tilt the pelvis—you do not want to use your buttocks, or grip the quadriceps. Do not raise your tail bone.

LIFTED FROGS

Aim:

To stretch the inside thighs.

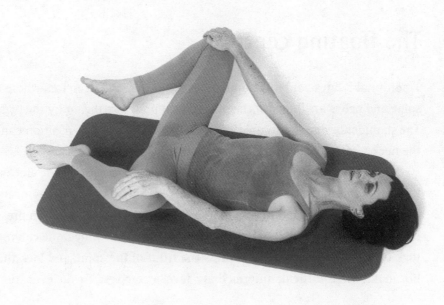

To start, lie in the constructive rest position, bending both legs up towards your chest so that your thighs are vertical above the pelvis, then lengthen your arms to place the hands on the inside of each knee.

Inhale. As you exhale engage your centre and then, gently press knees apart and towards the floor stretching your inside thighs. Ensure that your lower legs are relaxed and that the feet part, thus giving a more effective stretch. Inhale as you relax and bring the legs together with the feet relaxed.

Repeat 6 to 8 times.

Visualisation:

You are opening a book; your pelvis is the spine of the book, the legs are the covers.

Points of caution:

Take care not to arch the lower back off the floor. Let the weight of the legs and arms do most of the work while the breathing muscles steady the pelvis.

31 The floating centre

Traditional Pilates contains numerous shoulder bridge exercises where the lower spine and pelvis are lifted off the mat and supported in the air by the legs and feet. The shoulder bridge is also used in yoga. Unfortunately this position can overload the neck and strain the back unless done very carefully.

Many exercise teachers and some Pilates instructors use pelvic clocks, tilts and lifts, all involving some form of the shoulder bridge, as beginning or basic exercises. They can be found in other movement systems and are often prescribed by other body work professionals. I feel that the ease with which one can unwittingly tuck the pelvis, squash and compress the front of the spine and lock the anterior hip make these difficult intermediate-level exercises. To do even the simplest shoulder bridge beneficially requires a very good muscle recruitment pattern that is too hard for most beginners.

That said, supporting the centre in mid air is good for the body—after all, it is similar to what we do when we stand up, but in a different plane. The almost upside-down position of the shoulder bridge—with the shoulders down and the hips up in the air—enables us to challenge the shoulder girdle and connect it with the centre. It also helps to gain suppleness and balance through the lower and mid spine in a different way.

The pelvis is controlled by the abdominal muscles, lower back and hips, buttock muscles and upper leg muscles. It is the interface between our upright locomotor system and our prime postural supporting muscles. Suspending the centre between the feet and the shoulders helps to develop a feeling of space between the joints of the spine and lengthen our centre, if done with precision and awareness. Care needs to be taken so that the major buttock muscles do not overwork and the upper psoas muscle become braced.

COCCYX CURL TO BRIDGE LIFT

Aim:

To lengthen the space between the ribs and the pelvis. This is a good way of lengthening the lower spine, connecting with the centre, and using the hamstrings

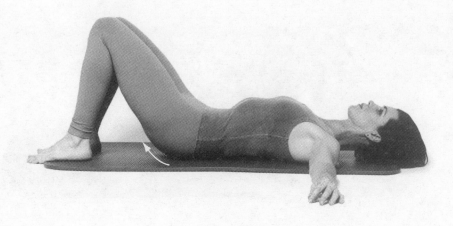

and deep buttock muscles with the hip flexors lengthened.

Coccyx curl

To start, lie in constructive rest position with the feet
parallel and hip width apart, arms by your sides.

Inhale and check neutral spine. As you exhale, press
down through the feet (particularly the toes) and slowly
curl up the tailbone. Lift and lengthen from the base of
the spine so that your coccyx rises away from the floor.
The lumbar spine remains on the floor. Inhale and return
to neutral spine.

Repeat 6 times.

Points of caution:

Take care not to over-tuck the pelvis. Try not to shorten
the distance between the pubic bone and the waist; keep
the centre elongated.

If you are comfortable with the coccyx curl and can
support your centre without gripping the outside
buttock muscles, progress to the shoulder bridge.

Bridge lift

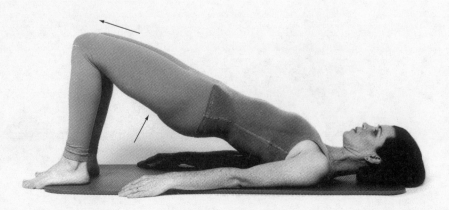

To start, lie in constructive rest position, as for the coccyx curl. Inhale, and connect with the soles of the feet. Exhale and, beginning with your coccyx, curl up your spine, away from the floor, lifting one vertebra at a time until you are resting evenly between the feet and the shoulders with the waist and spine lengthened. Inhale, remaining in the lifted position, then exhale and slowly uncurl to the floor and down to neutral spine.

Repeat 6 times.

Visualisation:

Think of massaging the spine off the floor, stretching the spine out and reaching the knees away. Imagine your spine is a hammock suspended evenly between your feet and shoulders.

Points of caution:

Take care not to part the knees as you lift up. Do not let the weight of the body fall only on the shoulders, but keep the feet and legs active with weight on the feet. Do not pinch your buttock muscles tightly together.

Variations:

When you are very comfortable with this exercise you can progress to a single leg lift. Stay in the bridge position and gently lift one leg off the floor in the bent position; the back of the supporting leg will work very hard.

BUTTOCK STRETCH

Aim:

To stretch the deeper bottom muscles.

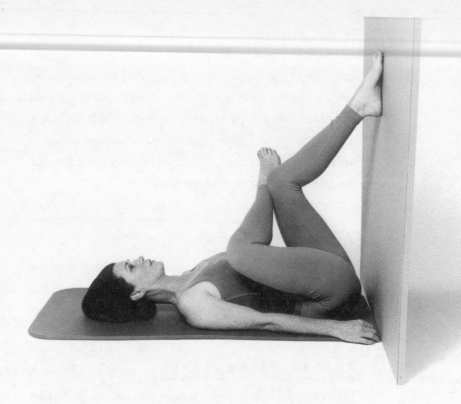

To start, lie down with your body on the floor close to a wall at right angles with the feet and legs extended, resting up against the wall. Cross one leg over the thigh at the ankle and gently bend the leg that is resting against the wall. This will bring the crossed leg towards your body. Continue to bring the bent leg down the wall until you feel a stretch in the back upper thigh and bottom of the crossed leg. Pause in the gently stretching position, inhale. Then exhale and lengthen your coccyx down into the floor to increase the stretch.

Repeat stretches for 6 breaths on one side, change legs and repeat on other side.

Visualisation:

Your coccyx is lengthening toward the floor while the

thigh of the crossed leg reaches away in the opposite direction.

Points of caution:

Take care to keep the hips square and the coccyx resting
... Do not push the crossed leg away from the

... es of the

... er muscles that attach to our neck
... and levator scapula are very often
... uscle that runs along the top of the
... ne, such as alternate arms over head
... idea of how to properly use those

... arms you need to hold the shoulder
... ine. You need to achieve a feeling of
... rmpit and side of the body, working
... res minor. The back of the top of the
... ur body, tend to be ignored in most
... the back of the thigh and the inside
... d by adjacent, easier to use, powerful
... rea properly improve its appearance,
... duced or even avoided.
... ce and effort, try sitting upright, then
... to the floor by your side, relaxing the
... owards the neck; now, staying there,
press the arm down and lift the body, using the armpit muscles. Your neck and head should move away from your shoulder and you should feel taller.

Upper body strength

MERMAID

Aim:

To work the upper body without overusing the upper shoulder muscles. This exercise focuses on upper body and shoulder girdle strength and control, which helps to sustain the range of movement of the arms, and oblique abdominal work.

To start, sit upright on the mat, with the legs bent and tucked in to one side, feet lengthened, sitting on one hip, with your arms down by your sides.

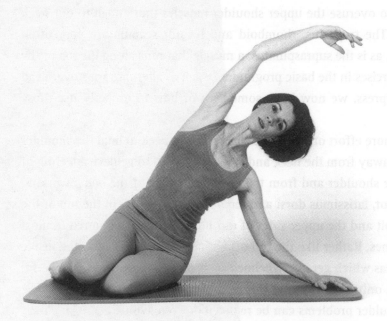

Inhale. As you exhale, slide the hand on the side you are sitting along the floor and away from your bent legs. Rest your body weight on that arm, keeping your shoulder down in alignment. With a lengthened spine reach the other arm over your head and stretch sideways. Inhale using your obliques. Draw the body back to centre and bring the raised arm down to the floor. As you return to sitting upright, exhale and reach the other arm overhead. You will not be able to bend very far as you cannot move the hip you are sitting on. Inhale, and return to the upright posture.

Repeat 6 times on each side.

Visualisation:

Reach your arm as far away from the opposite hip as possible, like a mermaid sitting on a rock and dipping her hand to the waves.

Points of caution:

Take care to only reach sideways, do not bend forward. Relax the neck and upper shoulders.

Variation:

When you are strong enough, bend the supporting arm down to the elbow as the other arm comes over your head.

SIDE PUSH UP

Aim:

To strengthen the armpit muscles and the front of the chest (the pectorals) and the back of the top of the arm (the triceps).

To start, lie on your side with the legs together, slightly bent up, the lower arm bent up across the chest and that hand resting on the upper shoulder. Place the

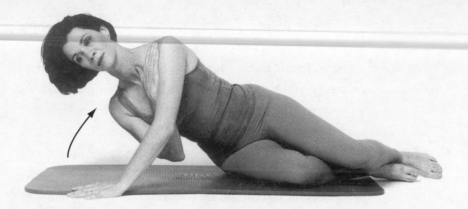

upper hand on the floor in front of your chest, palm down.

Begin with an inhale and connect with the palm to the floor. As you exhale press down into your palm, straightening the front arm and lifting your body with your upper side abdominal muscles and the muscles at the back of the arm in a slight spiral so that the chest opens away from the arm slightly. To complete the alignment of the spine look slightly down towards the hand on the floor.

Repeat 5 times on each side.

Visualisation:

You are pushing the floor away from your lower shoulder.

Points of caution:

Take care not to bring your shoulder to your ear. Keep the shoulder of the working side open by pressing the muscles at the back of the armpit down the side of the body towards the floor. Keep your legs relaxed and still.

33 From the ground up

Many people think that feet are there 'just to stop the legs from fraying', but there is a lot more to feet than that! In some body work professions there is a degree of awareness that foot problems and some lower back problems are connected. The usual remedy is to place orthotics in the shoes, but for most problems inserting arch supports is only a stopgap remedy at best. Unless the feet can improve their function, the short-term gain from orthotic inserts is lost when the muscles of the foot allow the arch support to take over their work completely. If the foot muscles themselves are not strengthened long term, loss of muscle function will not only continue, but usually worsen.

The feet are made up of many small variably shaped bones that fit together like a jigsaw puzzle in the shape of several archways, like a long, complex barrel vault. The bones remain closely in alignment only because the ligaments, tendons and muscles hold them together. Unless the muscles remain toned the arches will jam up or collapse. The pressures on the feet are enormous. Gravity and body weight constantly press down through the ankle onto the arches when we are standing. When we are moving, the dynamic action of the foot means it has to sustain a variety of impacts and forces. Some of the problems associated with retraining the feet stem from misunderstandings of the way that important foot muscles work.

The muscles that travel only across the foot, that start and finish in the foot are called intrinsic foot muscles; the muscles that start in the foot and travel across the ankle and up the lower leg are called extrinsic foot muscles. The extrinsic foot muscles are larger and longer than the intrinsic foot muscles. Many problems arise from the overuse and misuse of the extrinsic foot muscles and the underuse of the intrinsic foot muscles. Very often the intrinsic foot muscles are dismissed as only playing a static role in movement and arch support, when they are actually vital in assisting the foot to push off and propel the body in any upright movement, as well as affecting posture.

Some of this misunderstanding is due to the fact that it is easier to find and use the bigger extrinsic muscles and frustrating and difficult to find and use the smaller intrinsic muscles. Unfortunately, since we spend so much time on our feet, they are one of the hardest parts of the body to retrain. They do not get much rest but are continually jarred and subjected to impact as we move about. They are also usually most distant from our awareness.

One common problem is flat feet or pronation, when the arch of the foot flattens towards the floor. This may be structural or functional. Functional flat feet occur when the arches of the feet collapse because of the way they are used. This can cause severe problems, not just in the foot and ankle, but in the effect it has on leg and pelvic alignment, can end up causing back problems. Imagine a longbow with the string loose—the bow looses its curve, strength and resilience. By exercising the muscles of the arch underneath the foot we can improve the tone and spring of the 'bow', the arch of the foot. Exercising the muscles between the big toe and the heel can help reduce the discomfort of flat feet and recover the tone of the arch.

Exercising the feet not only improves foot muscle strength and function, it also helps our ability to keep our balance, recover from stumbles, avoid falls and improve our posture. Often it is only the calf muscles and the shin muscle (tibialis anterior) that work hard, but the side muscles of the lower leg (peroneals and tibialis posterior) also play an important role in ankle support. These muscles also attach to the underneath of the foot and therefore assist in arch stability. When the foot is moved upwards in dorsiflexion or pointed downwards in plantar flexion, the sliding hinge of the ankle needs to be kept aligned so that the toes do not turn out or in. There should be a straight line between the second toe and the middle of the ankle.

The feet and lower limbs are also a very important vascular pump. When we exercise the feet we increase arterial blood supply down the legs, which in turn improves the ability of the venous (used) blood to return to the heart. This dramatically assists lower limb circulation and reduces ankle swelling and blood pooling.

I advise clients that it takes a minimum of two years to retrain the feet. It is especially important to be very precise when working the feet. These exercises are vital for anyone who jogs, runs, plays squash or tennis, or who has flat or pronating feet or bunions.

It is best to start warming up the feet lying down when they are carrying no weight. Some of the later exercises are slightly weight bearing as the muscles need resistance to improve in strength. The Pilates principles of precision and persistence are particularly important with retraining feet as this area (along with the pelvic floor) is very slow to re-educate.

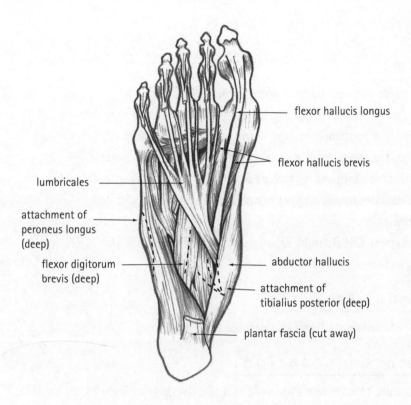

flexor hallucis longus

flexor hallucis brevis

lumbricales

attachment of
peroneus longus
(deep)

flexor digitorum
brevis (deep)

abductor hallucis

attachment of
tibialius posterior (deep)

plantar fascia (cut away)

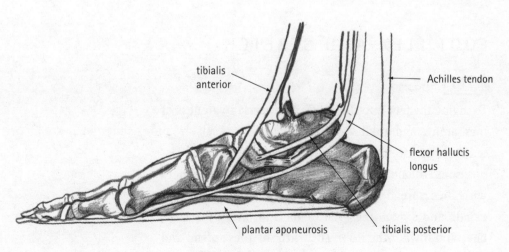

tibialis
anterior

Achilles tendon

flexor hallucis
longus

plantar aponeurosis

tibialis posterior

The anatomy of the foot

FOOT CIRCLES

Aim:

To warm up and connect with the feet.

To start, lie in a supported rest position or with your legs on a footstool or low chair with the feet relaxed. Circle the feet. Inhale as the feet come toward your shins, trace large slow circles down toward the floor as you exhale. Inhale as you bring your toes towards your knees.

Repeat this 8 times in one direction, then circle the feet in the other direction.

Visualisation:

You are stirring a bowl of porridge with your toes.

Points of caution:

Take care to only use your feet and not move your legs.

Variation:

You can also do this exercise sitting on a chair.

FOOT FLEX AND STRETCH

Aim:

To divide the feet into their different parts; awareness of toes, arches and ankle.

To start, lie in either of the above supported rest positions. Inhale. Stretch the feet up towards the knees with toes spread apart, then, keeping the toes back, exhale and stretch the arch of the foot away from the knee and toward the floor, still with the toes spread and lifted. Then stretch the toes away from the knee as you

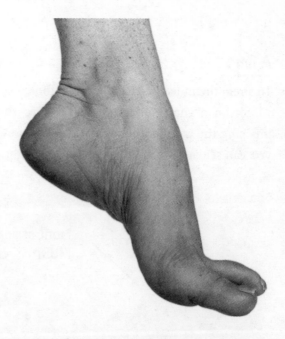

would point your foot. Inhale and lift the toes up to the ceiling, then bring the rest of the foot back so that your feet are flexed up to the ceiling, keeping alignment through your feet to your knees.

Repeat 8 times with both feet.

Visualisation:

Your feet are as mobile as your hands as they wave through the air.

Variation:

This exercise is surprisingly hard to do. If you find it difficult to move both feet together, exercise one foot at a time.

The next two exercises can be done at any time and do not need to be included in the full programme.

SITTING TOES AND ARCHES

Aim:

To strengthen the muscles under the foot.

Sit on a chair so that your feet are comfortably touching the ground and are parallel. Lean over so that you can see your feet, putting a bit of weight on them.

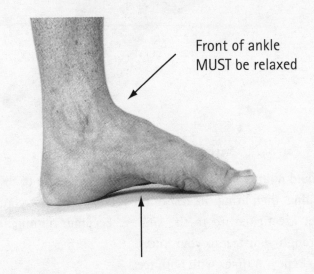

Front of ankle
MUST be relaxed

Have a good look at them, check that they are aligned with the second toes and middle of the ankles parallel. Inhale. Then lengthen and spread your toes, lifting them up off the floor so that there is space between each toe. Exhale as you press your toes into the floor without scrunching or curling them up. Press the big toe down and try to get the middle toe joints to lengthen out. Elevate the short arch and across the lower foot to lift the ends of the metatarsals. At the same time lift the long arches of the foot upward, drawing your toes towards your heels with the arch muscles of the feet.

Repeat 8 times.

Visualisation:

You have small balloons under your arches that are being inflated as you elevate your arches. You have suckers under your toes, like the tentacles of an octopus, holding onto the ground as you lift your arches.

Points of caution:

It is crucial *not* to use the front foot-to-shin muscle (tibialis anterior) that crosses over the front of the ankle. Only connect with and use the muscles under the foot. This is very hard to do.

TENNIS BALL MASSAGE

Aim:

This is a useful stretch to encourage relaxation of the plantar muscles, the muscles under the arch of the foot.

To start, stand up holding onto a wall for support and balance. Place a tennis ball under the foot, near the heel. Inhale. Press down and move the foot back slowly as you exhale, massaging the arch. As the ball goes towards the front of the foot, pause with it under the ball of the foot and inhale. Then exhale, press and roll the ball back as your foot moves forward.

This exercise can be done any time. It is particularly good at the end of a long day.

34 Improving heart rate, circulation and endurance

Aerobic activity is exercise that uses the ordinary supply of oxygen as the body's fuel. Our everyday life is primarily performed with our aerobic energy system. These are the ordinary gentle movements of life up to moderately paced movement or exercise. Your heart rate may increase slightly and you may feel a bit warm, but aerobic movement can be continued without pause or stopping to rest, as energy is continually supplied via the reoxygenated blood we pump around our bodies.

By improving the use and efficiency of our aerobic system we can sustain our fitness, endurance and energy needs.

Anaerobic processes are forced into action when the ordinary oxygen supply is not enough, using glycogen which is stored in the muscles. Anaerobic exercise tends to be short term, such as lifting a huge weight, or running as fast as possible. We cannot continue the activity for long. We need to stop and rest to give the body time to remove the waste products created. The anaerobic system uses unsustainable effort. Our heart rate increases enormously and muscles, joints and ligaments tend to be placed under pressure.

Sustaining moderate effort pushes the boundary between the aerobic system and the anaerobic system and allows us to increase our fitness without injuring ourselves. Practicing the complete programme in this book will improve your general fitness and health using your aerobic energy system.

The Pilates method also assists in improving and sustaining good circulation, by ensuring that all the muscles of the body are exercised equally. The modern method particularly helps the lower leg and foot circulation with the introduction of a range of foot exercises.

When we think of improving fitness for ourselves we need to be aware of our basic body type (ectomorph, mesomorph or endomorph). Doing what we enjoy often means doing what comes easily. But to really challenge ourselves, doing a bit of what does not come naturally is very important. If you are basically an ectomorph, endurance work and de-stressing will be important, if you are more of a mesomorph you will probably need to improve flexibility. The endomorph needs to work on the aerobic threshold to challenge their excellent ability to store food!

The basic programme will not challenge your heart as the gentle flow of movement stays completely within the aerobic system. The intermediate programme can improve your aerobic threshold and moderately challenge the cardiovascular system. When the exercises are mastered you will be able to increase the pace at which you do them, pausing only briefly between each. The better you do the exercises the more work you will achieve.

35 Connecting basic to intermediate

The full at-home programme

The basic exercise programme and the intermediate can be merged to form one complete programme of about 45 minutes. You can also make up a variety of programmes using the basic programme as a foundation and adding a few exercises from the intermediate programme to create a shorter programme—from a brief 15 minutes to 25 or 30 minutes.

Keeping up a regular pattern of exercise is the key to good health. Look at how often we eat, clean our teeth, sleep, wake and get dressed. We do not have much of a problem understanding that doing those things daily is ordinary and normal—we rarely think that we should not do those things—but what about exercise?

From school age onward exercise becomes restricted and regimented; something to avoid or ritually overdo (sport). Moderate regular exercise keeps us healthy and fit. Exercise is good for the mind as well as the body. It lets us have mental space, lets us relax the mind; it reduces depression and encourages good hormone production. It helps us keep our bones strong and our heart and lungs working.

When preparing to exercise, give yourself time to follow through with a complete sequence of exercises to connect with all the body. Lie down on your mat in a supported rest position and mentally go through the principles and connect with your body, letting go of tension and outside distractions.

Concentrate and

Focus **Awareness** on your body

Check **Alignment**

Use **Breathing** to connect with neutral spine, then

Find your **Centre**

Then begin with the gentle warm up from the basic programme; lie on your back and begin.

Breathing, find neutral spine

initiate moving with **Precision**

And **Coordination**

Always **Lengthening**

Persist in your practice

Combined Exercise sequence

Basic programme   Intermediate programme

Supine:

head rolls, shoulder shrugs

single leg slides, single knee side

single arm floats progress to

    alternate arms, arm slides

Prone:

stomach lifts

diamond press, single leg lift   sphinx to single leg flick

Lateral:

breathing, clams, single leg lift   side double leg lift

Supine:

double knee press

4-point kneeling:

breathing, progress to cat stretch   4-point kneeling plank

kneeling hamstrings stretch

rest position

Intermediate progressions

	1	*2*

Supine:

1	2
if you have back or neck problems do not do *curl ups*, straight and diagonal	curl ups
	single leg stretches
	single leg circles

Supine:

1	2
If you have short hamstrings *sit on a chair*:	hamstring stretch with towel
seated on a chair spine stretch	progress to spine stretch on mat
seated on feet mid spine extension	progress to sitting on mat
	mid spine extension
	rolling (only if doing the spine stretch and extension on a mat)
seated on a chair the saw	progress to the saw on the mat
seated on a chair the spine twist	progress to sitting on mat
	spine twist
upper body supported side leg flick	progress to elbows

Supine:

1	2
pelvic floor lifts	pelvic floor lifts progress to elevators
pillow squeeze	
lifted frogs	
coccyx lift to bridge lift	progress to bridge lift with single leg lift
buttock stretch	

Side sit: | mermaid

Lateral: | side push ups

Supine:

feet

185

Lie on your side to finish your exercise programme on the mat, and conclude with the arm openings and stretch and yawn from the basic programme. Rest on the mat for a moment before you roll on your side to sit up, and slowly stand.

This final exercise should only be attempted once you have felt comfortable with the previous exercises for some time, and only if you have no back problems.

THE STANDING ROLL DOWN

Aim:

Assists in transition from standing to lying or vice versa comfortably articulate through the spine.

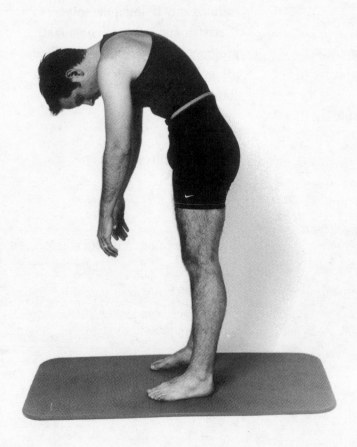

To start, stand with the feet hip-width apart with the body lengthened upright. Slowly curl forward and down as you exhale, articulating through the spine one vertebra at a time. Let the head and arms hang down, relaxed, with the knees slightly bent. Inhale, relaxing down completely, then exhale as you slowly uncurl to stand upright.

First the head and then the back should curl down. The pelvis should release forward only as the lower spine uncurls, with the top part tilting over and slightly towards the floor. Do not bounce or force your body down in to this position. Inhale. Then exhale and uncurl.

Repeat this 3 times, standing up tall and connected with all your body.

This concludes the exercises for the complete intermediate home programme.

Exercise as part of life

Incorporate movement in your regular life. You can do bits of movement, with awareness of posture and breathing intermittently during the day. Do not be fanatical, just persistent. Pelvic floor exercises, for example, can be done any time, anywhere, once you have mastered them lying down. You can do them in the car at stop lights, standing at the bus stop, or while sitting at the computer. Foot exercises can be done while you sit watching TV, or listening to music, or at your desk.

As well as finding time to exercise regularly for a consistent minimum 20 or 30 minutes three times per week, going to a reputable, experienced Pilates studio at least once a week will help you stay on track and allow you to try more advanced work safely.

Part IV

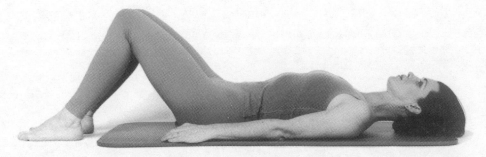

Ongoing care

In this final section I will discuss how we learn to look after ourselves over the long term, and look at ways to sustain fitness using the Pilates method without causing injuries. I also include a few suggestions on avoiding and caring for injuries. Even though the Pilates method is primarily practiced lying down, we can directly and safely apply it to everyday life and activities. Modern Pilates helps us to inhabit the whole of our bodies, for long-term fitness and health. As you become more connected with your body you may begin to notice more aches or tight bits. This is not unusual; one of the first things modern Pilates does is to help connect the body as you continue to practice. Gradually your body will respond and connect with better senses, sharpened awareness, improved movement with grace and ease; but there is no instant fix. It is only with perseverance that long-term changes happen.

Movement is the foundation of life. Our muscles are imbued with sensation, memories and feelings; not just the feeling of hardness or softness, weakness or strength, but with a broad range of complex emotions. Be aware of this, and recognise that body and mind are completely linked. To look after one, we need to look after the other. It is the interaction between the two that makes us uniquely human.

36 Body habits

Our own body habits of movement develop over time. They come from our genetic makeup and are constantly influenced by our life experiences. It is not just what we do (physically) that affects our body. All our mental and emotional activities also impinge one way or another upon it. Our mind is part of our body and vice versa. Life experience influences body movement patterns, which in turn affects how we respond to our next life experience.

The practice of modern Pilates truly reflects this understanding of the entwining of sense, perception, cognition, emotion, motion and stillness, growth, stasis and maturity. The sense of the passage of time is most honestly reflected in the body, which carries with it a history of self that is unsullied by the mind's ability to forget or screen out memories of past events. Just as physical scars and injuries fade but never entirely vanish, so may feelings and memories become integrated into various layers of our posture—they are hard to tease out, but they are all there.

Emotions do not just reside in the head; they saturate the body's musculature, and the viscera. How often do we have a gut feeling? Or get butterflies in the stomach? When do we go weak at the knees? Grit our teeth in rage or determination?

Senses, feelings and emotions dwell within the body and are given outward expression by it. The interpretation of an experience may be retained in the mind but the action and reaction remain anchored in the soft tissue of our muscles and fascia, and in the movement patterns and habits that we develop in the light of our experiences.

Having a good awareness of our bodies allows us to look after ourselves. With a good connection between mind and body we reduce our vulnerability to injury, and are less likely to be shocked or let down by the body. Just as we engage our minds we need to engage and respect our bodies. The expression 'use it or lose it' applies to both.

How should we look after our bodies

Repeating the same thought pattern or body movement, mindlessly, for many years does not equal years of experience bringing understanding and maturity. That is just habit, which is not associated with growth, or finding different ways to solve 'binds' or problems. The body and its muscles are part of our 'historical record'— our present day's actions are founded on yesterday's experiences. Just as we can become stuck in a thought pattern, so we can get stuck in a movement pattern.

Connecting, understanding, unwinding and exploring different movement possibilities in the deeper postural layers is the most direct way of challenging bind and 'stuckness'. It is important to go gently when re-educating the body, as connecting with the unsorted past can at times be shocking, but handled well, the interplay between body memory and recollection can produce the most extraordinary maturity and growth. It can, however, be very distressing learning about one's self in isolation without a support structure and a way of picking up the pieces, so any in-depth exploration needs to be very well supervised.

Modern Pilates is a way of moving safely and comfortably, in all possible dimensions, with resilience and emotional responsiveness. Initially we take away the direct downward tug of gravity on our postural muscles in the upright position, and lie down to re-educate muscular habits. We connect with our breathing and internal sensations. Then we lengthen and strengthen those muscles to enable our bodies to function well, whether we are standing, sitting, bending, walking, reaching and grasping, or leaping.

The Pilates method works against the changes of ageing, to lessen the decline in body skills over the years. The modern Pilates method helps to sustain a youthful posture, and resists the decline of lower limb and foot strength and co-ordination. Thinking and feeling are practised as an integral part of the method which helps the mind to remain alert.

Because the Pilates method is tailored to individuals' changing needs, it is a particularly good form of sustainable exercise for those going through any of life's major changes, for example, preparing for pregnancy. When a woman becomes pregnant, not only is it the start of a new life but her body undergoes specific changes. Hormones are released that effect ligaments and joints, making them more relaxed and therefore overflexible. Regular exercising with modern Pilates supports good muscle tone and reduces the potential of overtaxing lax joints. The pelvic floor exercises are particularly beneficial, both ante- and post-natal.

37 Exercise sequencing and types of learning

Learning anything new takes time and energy. With persistence, our awareness improves and translates to physical understanding. That improved physical ability links back into the sensory systems and our mind. Our physical, mental, emotional and sensory abilities interact with each other to broaden and deepen our knowledge and physical competence. We grow.

The way we learn varies depending on our ability to absorb and retain information. Some of us learn more easily via demonstration or by listening, copying, direct guidance with touch, visualisation. Some of us retain new information quickly in terms of shape, images, rhythm, coordination, feeling, or focus on specific details. Our approach to learning can vary greatly from person to person; think how one friend has the ability to recall numbers, or how you may have the ability always to find your way. You may find that you remember the exercises more easily if you exercise to music. You may want to make a tape recording of the exercise names, or make a written list. You may find that you do better with a good Pilates method practitioner, who will use a variety of instruction methods to find which is most relevant to you.

You yourself may work out specific ways of reminding your body how to move effectively. Whatever our particular skills, over time we digest and store and apply new ways of doing things. We all acquire body habits. We sit, tie our shoelaces, eat and drive a car in a particular, individual way. As you practise Pilates you may notice subtle changes indirectly—your friends seem to be getting shorter, lifting the shopping out of the car doesn't make your back ache, a social sport becomes easier, you walk places rather than automatically drive the car.

Changing the ways we move occurs very gradually, with occasional sudden spurts of improvement. We can initiate change unaided up to a point, but often supervision is needed to assist greater improvement or when we have an injury or other problem to deal with. Finding that you are very sore after a Pilates class probably means that you are working too hard—your body is not yet able to integrate efficient movement practice and has overused some muscles, hence the soreness. Advancing your movement abilities happens in fits and starts with practice over time. The ability to perceive time via change comes through comparing improvement or decay in the body's skills: 'I used to be able to touch my toes—I can now touch my toes'. Time is punctuated by such changes.

Exercise trees

I have tried to make this book informative and easy to follow. However, I know there is too much to digest in one go—there is too much to digest even in several goes. As you practise the exercises initially, re-read the appropriate description before you start each movement. Once you are happy with the general idea behind an exercise, move through the sequence, following the instructions as you work. Once you have established the sequence of movement and breathing, choose one aspect or principle of the exercise to focus on. As you work through the other exercises, continue to follow through on that principle. Use this chapter to develop your favourite way of sustaining learning.

I developed the idea of exercise trees as a learning and teaching tool when training teachers in the Pilates method. Using the image of a tree was a straightforward way of working out how to sequence any movement re-education programme. People found it much more interesting, and learned much faster, than using the usual limited linear model—'first do Exercise 1, then 2, then 3, etc.'. Re-educating the body is a huge task. We cannot do everything at once but relearning movement skills involves far more than just doing one thing at a time.

So I use the image of a tree to choose what to concentrate on and to help choose what to learn next. The tree image fits well with the process of modern Pilates—growth and change with stability and movement. The three-dimensionality, solidity and longevity of a large tree is important. Think of bending with the impact of life, not breaking, with the foundations or roots of the method supporting the central body of work and the branches providing the many variations and alternatives for sustaining fitness and health.

Following the model of the tree, we can work through the modern principles as we practise. Sometimes we struggle for a while till we get things connected and working in a better way. Then suddenly everything clicks into place—we unconsciously breathe from our centre, keeping better alignment, with beautifully coordinated movements and the correct muscles working from the centre.

The exercises themselves have a sequence that follows from the simplest movement toward the more complex, thus laying a foundation of solid building blocks to enable the body to more easily absorb and improve postural patterns by working from the deeper layers of residual posture and using the centre and lengthening. Following the basic programme you can move on to the intermediate programme, increasing the speed and complexity of movement for improved fitness and grace and economy of movement.

Often you will not have the time to do all the exercises. Doing some of them is fine. It is a good idea to vary the sequence of the exercises so the body does not habitually do one exercise after another.

You can create your own exercise trees. Begin with the gentle pre-Pilates exercises and increase the complexity and the range of movement; vary the load on your centre, and attend to the stabilisers by choosing different intermediate exercises. Ensure that you exercise the body in all the different positions: lying on your front, your back and your side.

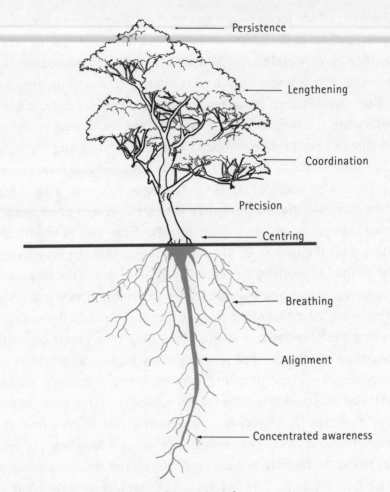

Modern Pilates principles

Persistence—physical repetitions over long periods of time—mental focus—
sustained grace and economy of movement
Lengthening—alignment centre—joints—precision—long, slender muscular
development
Coordination—precision—alignment—breathing—good balance—ease of movement
Precision—comes with awareness—alignment—breathing—centring—fine motor
control
Centring—supine—prone—lateral
Breathing—siphon—bellows—piston
Alignment—posture—torso/spine—head—limbs
Concentrated awareness—focused thinking and feeling—sensing

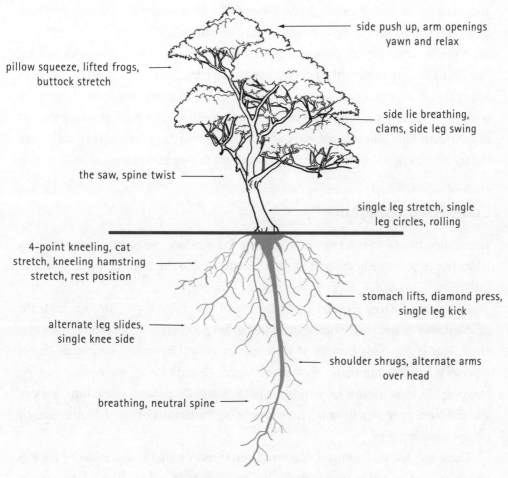

side push up, arm openings
yawn and relax

pillow squeeze, lifted frogs,
buttock stretch

side lie breathing,
clams, side leg swing

the saw, spine twist

single leg stretch, single
leg circles, rolling

4-point kneeling, cat
stretch, kneeling hamstring
stretch, rest position

stomach lifts, diamond press,
single leg kick

alternate leg slides,
single knee side

shoulder shrugs, alternate arms
over head

breathing, neutral spine

Examples of short intermediate sequence

Growth

Being able to coordinate with precision and work all the muscles of the body evenly with flowing movement and sustained concentration is a sign that you are ready to progress to new, more complex movements. Before you go on to another exercise, or a new variation, however, be aware of any commonly over-recruited muscles or tension. Sometimes a specific problem needs to be worked on not by challenging it directly but by increasing work with neighbouring muscles. Self-correction has its limitations, however. To progress to the more complex exercises, you need to be under experienced supervision in a reputable Pilates studio to avoid the risk of setting up the wrong muscle patterns.

When it comes to your posture, note that some internal postural muscles will not just be tight, but noticeably twitchy, when the main overused postural muscles relax. This is a good sign that you can move along to something new. Sometimes postural muscles are strong only in one prime position and weak through the rest of the range. First, allow incorrectly used postural muscles to relax, then train subsidiary or synergistic muscles, then go back and retrain postural muscles.

Combating boredom

The ability to progress varies enormously from person to person. Sometimes a wider range of movements and variations will have to be introduced on a similar skill level to avoid feelings of stuckness or boredom.

For many Pilates method instructors and practitioners of the method, the simplest way to overcome boredom is just to keep expanding the number of exercises. This is the 'let's do lots of different exercises' or 'more' syndrome—more repertory, more equipment, more resistance. Quantity can overcome quality, however. As long as you keep to the basics as a good general warm-up, you can add different exercises gradually, always being conscious of the different muscle groups working well.

There are many other pre-Pilates and variations on traditional Pilates exercises which are not included in this book, but are taught in a qualified Pilates studio. You can add any variation you have been taught to this intermediate programme, but only when you feel comfortable doing the basic exercises at home.

38 Strong but unsafe: traditional exercises to avoid

When we put huge amounts of effort into a movement or series of movements our attention tends to focus on keeping the effort going by forcing the body. With high degrees of strain or force, however, we lose sensory connection or specific muscle ability in the attempt to focus that effort. If we try to do a very difficult exercise before we have established a foundation for it through the simpler exercises, the messages of effort are sent to the strongest muscles, the most overused muscles. If we have not retrained the body to use specific muscles in a lengthened way, those strong muscles will bunch up in effort. The body cannot discriminate initially, which means that the more difficult and more complex exercises are easier to 'cheat' on—as the body tries to make very effortful shapes it uses all the muscles, locking and bracing joints. (Rather like a baby who reaches for and grasps an object arbitrarily at first, later refining how and what it grasps.)

It is very hard to be muscle-specific when using huge effort. Some of the traditional Pilates exercises which fall into the category of 'very effortful', are therefore unsafe to do until the appropriate strong muscle connections are established in our abdominals and other commonly underworked muscles. It is safer to build up to these more difficult exercises, but not attempt them first.

Traditional exercises

The signature Pilates exercise was 'the Hundred'. Pilates stated that the first exercise should be the Hundred, and that 'one should not attempt any other exercise till you have mastered that'. This complex exercise is fraught with difficulty for anyone of moderate fitness or with back/neck problems. Any double leg elevation in the supine position is risky, as the hip flexors tend to overwork and the lower back and neck can easily be strained and injured, the throat become tightened and breathing constricted. There are many modern modifications to the Hundred, but any exercise that requires you to have both legs raised off the ground, and your head and shoulders raised at the same time, is going to put huge

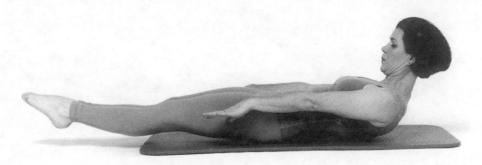

pressure on your lower back. This exercise should not be attempted in any form until your centre is very strong, and only if you have no back problems.

The Hundred can be approached as a breathing exercise or as an abdominal workout. The biomechanics are such that it does not just primarily exercise the abdominals. It is a whole body exercise that raises the heart rate and body temperature very fast—that is its beauty—but it does not exercise all muscles equally. The Hundred exercises the strong muscles of the front of the body while trying to make a fixed shape. The body recruits any muscles it can to create that shape. In some ways it is an easy exercise because we can lock the body in a slightly flexed position with the head up like a balanced banana. But since it is primarily done with the legs slightly turned out, with the spine heavily loaded, it is a very dangerous exercise, and should never be attempted until you have mastered control of your centre (which may take several years).

Many other traditional Pilates exercises like the double leg stretch and the teaser present serious problems, just like the Hundred, because both head and legs are raised at the same time. Please do not ever attempt these exercises on your own. They should not be taught at all until a very advanced level has been reached—and never right at the beginning of class.

The traditional exercises that start prone, on your stomach, and also elevate the upper body and both legs at the same time, such as the double leg kick (below) and the swan dive, require specific flexibility in the hip flexors and the ability comfortably to load extension of the lower back. Similarly to the Hundred, these exercises are very difficult to do without over-recruiting a small group of muscles and straining the lower back, and are likely to be dangerous for the beginner.

Any exercises done while resting the body's weight primarily on the neck and

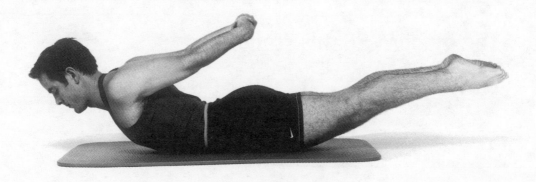

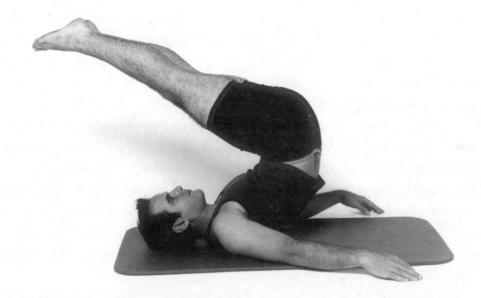

shoulders can cause problems for that region of our body. Exercises such as roll overs, the corkscrew (above) and the jack knife can cause neck injuries in anyone who has suffered an injury such as whiplash and in people whose neck area is not strong, and should never be attempted.

To attempt the complex intermediate and advanced Pilates exercises you need to be very fit and flexible. It is important also that you have no problems or injuries. Once you have mastered pre-Pilates and basic and intermediate exercises, the more complex work can be slowly added, *BUT*–this level of movement skill should only be attempted under careful supervision at a recognised Pilates method studio.

39 The modern Pilates studio

The equipment

The modern Pilates studio is usually equipped with floor mats and raised benches and various strange-looking pieces of equipment and machines. Joe Pilates was very good at inventing exercise equipment, from sliding beds (the universal reformer) to four-posted contraptions with metal springs (the Cadillac or trapeze table). A Pilates studio may resemble a mediaeval torture chamber or an S&M parlour with its curved, strange-shaped chairs, barrels, pillows and other foam shapes. The equipment may also include inflated balls (both small and very large), rubber tubing and bands, and a selection of modest free weights.

Joe Pilates developed his mat and floor exercises first. The universal reformer, and other machines like the Cadillac or trapeze table and the Wunda chair, use a variety of springs for variable load. The Pilates machines offer resistance and assistance, helping the exercising body keep good alignment, and assisting in centring and coordinating. The most popular apparatus, the universal reformer, is a sliding platform on rails with various springs for resistance work. You can lie, sit, kneel or stand on the reformer, using your legs and/or arms to move the platform under resistance.

The moderate resistance provided by the equipment improves the quality of sensation to that area and allows us to work harder. Some equipment, 'toys' such as the barrels, pillows, poles, and magic circle, assist the body to sustain shapes it otherwise may not be able to. Apart from adding variety they are only there to assist the client to connect with the right muscles and work them properly in a comfortable alignment.

The instructors

The most important thing about a professional Pilates studio is the instructors. They should be attentive, guiding you in your work, occasionally correcting movements. They should listen to your questions, offering thoughtful verbal advice and/or demonstrating and carefully guiding you with hands-on touch. They should offer just enough correction and help that you can improve without feeling pressured; they should provide a non-competitive relaxed environment.

The Pilates method is very 'touchy'. Pilates himself would press, hold, lift, poke, prod or pull any body part he felt needed to work more or have a better alignment. While modern instructors are mostly a little more circumspect about this hands-on approach, it is still not only a very useful way of being guided in your work, but also a good way of sensing and connecting with the body for yourself. Your hands have many nerves and can help you to connect with the rest

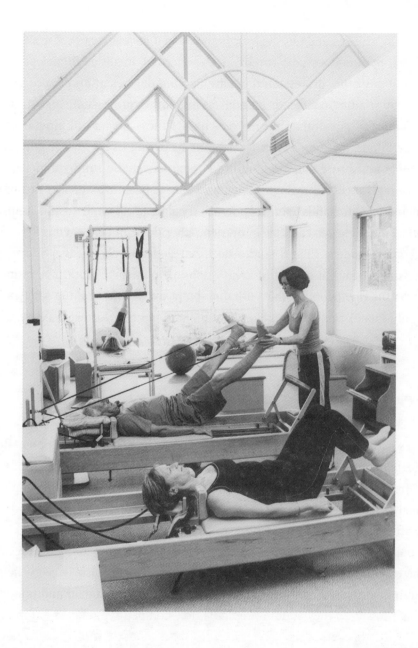

of your body; when you place your hands on a muscle you want to work more, the sensation of your hands can encourage the muscle underneath to engage. Some of what makes a good instructor is the quality of their hands-on skills. Touching needs to be done with subtlety, and a precision that is non-invasive though definite. The human body is extraordinarily resilient, and can cope with all sorts of stresses and physical strain, but if you have any sort of injury problem it is vital to attend a studio run by an experienced, qualified Pilates practitioner.

As in any other profession there are varying degrees of excellence. A two- or three-day training course, as an add-on to another profession, such as a human movement or physiotherapy degree, or a fitness leader's diploma, does *not* make a Pilates instructor. Equally, anyone behaving like a god or guru is worth avoiding. Make sure you are going to a reputable studio run by a member of an ethical registered professional association. Any form of exercise, in the wrong (undereducated) hands can be potentially damaging and unsafe. Improperly taught Pilates classes can cause injuries rather than prevent them.

A good modern Pilates studio does not depend only on the equipment for exercising, though it can be of great importance in some work. The prime focus is to get the client comfortable with their body, aware and working safely and able to apply Pilates principles to everyday life and to other forms of exercise.

40   The Pilates method and injury

Pilates can be of great benefit in a variety of health conditions. Because of the gentle non-impact nature of modern Pilates it is a very safe way of exercising after trauma or soft-tissue injury or to relieve chronic injury. Most importantly, a good practitioner can tailor the exercises to your specific needs, such as during and after pregnancy. Some long-term conditions can benefit from work with an experienced Pilates practitioner, such as some types of high blood pressure, asthma, diabetes, arthritis and osteoporosis. Modern Pilates can also be very helpful in resolving non-specific lower back problems and other joint pain and injuries.

Trauma

The best thing would be never to sustain an injury at all, but we all sustain various injuries over the course of a normal life. As children we frequently fall and bump ourselves, and our resilient bodies bounce back, most of the time. Occasionally we sustain serious injuries or become extremely ill, but mostly we recover well. Our body adapts to what we do to it from a very early age.

Gradually, as we get bigger and heavier, falls and other injuries begin to inflict more damage because impact increases with weight and speed. Even with severe injuries, if properly looked after and rested we can recover well. But if injuries are not looked after well and adequate recuperation not permitted, it may take a very long time to recover. During this process the body may develop compensatory habits of movement to avoid pain or re-injury: it adapts. We might stand mainly on one foot, or tilt the head slightly, hunch a shoulder up, reduce the range of movement in an arm or leg.

We often incorporate these adaptations so that they become part of our ordinary posture even when the injury is completely repaired. Accidents or sudden acute injuries cannot be avoided but how we look after them is important. They may turn into chronic injuries or the adaptations we make for the initial injury may set us on the path to further injury.

Overuse or chronic injury

Many chronic injuries develop surreptitiously. If we repeatedly overtax an area of the body without allowing rest and recuperation, the body gradually finds continuing with the repeated overwork very difficult. The overworked area becomes strained and sustains pain and sends messages to the brain to stop and rest, which we may ignore. If we refuse to listen to the body we can develop chronic injuries that may last months or even years. Occasionally they improve, but more often the injury becomes progressively worse. Finally we have to stop whatever it is we can no longer do comfortably, perhaps typing at a computer, long distance running or playing golf.

Compensatory patterns may fail when we are not warmed up or fit enough, when we are already overstrained from other activities or are tense due to unsorted and unexpressed emotion. Further compensatory patterns are then created, to avoid pain or discomfort. We may go numb in the injured area. This can work for a while, but if the pattern of compensation becomes fixed or out of balance, serious long-term problems may arise.

Listen to your body, be aware of when it is overworked, and give it a chance to unwind and recuperate. Being familiar with your body includes knowing your body type, and being aware that the different body types do not just reflect shape, muscle tone and flexibility but also emotional resilience or brittleness. Your metabolic rate relates to how frequently your fight and flight reflex is activated, as well as your ability to relax.

We all have a particularly vulnerable part of the body that reacts to stress. You might suffer repeated strains in the wrist. You might ask yourself what makes me feel 'h'arm less? Do you gnaw away at problems, unable to let them go, and suffer jaw and tooth problems? These things are part of our uniqueness, but it is not good to be ruled by them. It is healthy to reduce our vulnerability to repeat injuries or chronic pain.

Soft-tissue injury

In the short term, straight after sustaining a soft-tissue injury, it is very important to rest, ice and elevate the injured part. Continue to do this while the injury-site remains swollen. When it is comfortable to do so, beginning with small gentle movements which cause no pain, exercise gently to keep the area from stiffening up. If the injury is severe it is important to see an appropriate medical practitioner for possible further treatment.

Pilates is a particularly good form of exercise when you have an injury such as bruising, a simple sprain or muscle strain. You can rest the injured area while still working the non-injured areas of the body. Pilates is good after the acute phase, or when the pain is no longer severe, for example with any tendonitis and non-specific back strains. Good Pilates also substantially aids recovery in post-acute rehabilitation after various operations.

At a reputable experienced Pilates studio the instructors can look at what weaknesses or restricted tight body habits have contributed to your chronic injury and work at reducing the risk of the injury happening again.

Disclaimer

Always check with your doctor before starting any exercise programme if you are diabetic, have high blood pressure or severe asthma, suffer from other chronic health problems, are extremely unfit and/or very overweight, or over 55 years old.

Various medical problems may improve over time with careful management in a good Pilates programme. But it is very important to note, particularly in association with any back problem: any loss in sensation, change in sensation, loss of function or tingling in the lower limbs, tripping, or a dropped foot, as these are signs that possible nerve damage is occurring. If this happens you need to seek medical opinions for further diagnosis and/or treatment. Pilates is *not* a cure-all and the more advanced exercises can be quite dangerous if not taught properly.

Bibliography

Calais-Germaine, B. (1993) *Anatomy of Movement*, Eastland Press Inc. USA

Chaiton, L. (ed.) (1996) *Journal of Bodywork and Movement Therapy (JMBT)*, Churchill-Livingston, Edinburgh

Encyclopaedia Britannica (2000), CD Rom

Fitt, Sally (1988) *Dance Kinesiology*, Schirmer Books USA

Franklin, Eric (1996) *Dynamic Alignment Through Imagery*, Human Kinetics, Champaign, IL

Friedman, P. and Eisen, G. (1980) *Pilates Method of Physical and Mental Conditioning*, Doubleday & Co., New York

Gallagher, S. and Kryzanowski, R. (1999) *The Pilates Method of Body Conditioning*, Bainbridge Books, Philadephia, PA

Hinkle, Carla Z. *Anatomy and Movement*

Johnson, Don J. (ed.) (1995) *Bone, Breath and Gesture*, North Atlantic Books, Berkeley, CA

Kapit, W. and Elson, L. (1993) *The Anatomy Coloring Book* (2nd edn), Addison Wesley, New York

Kendall, F.R., McCreary, E.K. and Provance, P.G. (1993) *Muscles: Testing and Function* (4th edn), Williams & Wilkins, Baltimore, MD

Latey, P. (1979) *Muscular Manifesto*, Osteopathic Publishing

Latey, P. (1999) 'Feelings, muscles, movement' *JBMT*, Churchill-Livingstone, Edinburgh

Martini, F., Bartholomew, E. and Welch, K. (1997) *Applications Manual of Essential Anatomy and Physiology*, Prentice Hall, USA

Mullan, H. (1999) *The World Encyclopaedia of Boxing*, Carlton Books, London

Myers, T. (1999) 'Spiral anatomy trains', *JBMT*, Churchill-Livingstone, Edinburgh & video

Nathan, Bevis (1999) *Touch and Emotion in Manual Therapy*, Churchill-Livingstone, Edinburgh

Pilates, J.H. ([1934] 1988) *Your Health*, Presentation Dynamics Inc., Nevada

Pilates, J.H. and Miller, W. ([1945] 1998) *Return to Life Through Contrology*, Presentation Dynamics Inc, Nevada

Platzer, W. (1992) *The Locomotor System* (4th edn), Theime Medical, USA

Porterfield, J.J. and DeRosa, C. (1991) *Mechanical Low Back Pain: Perspectives in Functional Anatomy*, Saunders W.B. Co., USA

Robinson, L. and Thompson, G. (1997) *Body Control the Pilates Way*, Macmillan, UK

Shorter Oxford Dictionary (1973), Oxford University Press, Oxford

Sparrow, L. (1994) *Amazing Mind–Body Machines*, Yoga Journal, USA

The Method Forum (previously The Pilates Forum) (1991–2000) *Journal of the Physicalmind Institute* (previously The Institute for the Pilates Method), Santa Fe, NM

The Physicalmind Institute (1993–95) Videos of J.H. Pilates and Eve Gentry, Santa Fe, NM

Todd, Mabel E. ([1937] 1968) *The Thinking Body*, Dance Horizons, Princeton Book Co., USA

Townsend, D. (ed.) (1994) *The New Penguin Dictionary of Modern History 1789–1945*, Penguin Books, UK

Weinbeck, J. ([1941] 1986) *Functional Anatomy in Sports*, Year Book Medieval Publishers Inc., Chicago, IL

Wide, A. (1906) *Medical and Orthopedic Gymnastics*, Funk & Wagnalls, New York

Winsor, M. (1999) *The Pilates Powerhouse*, Perseus Books, New York

Index